Unlocking the Value of NPs and PAs:

INCREASE REVENUE AND CREATE A HEALTHY AND THRIVING PRACTICE WITH MIDLEVEL PROVIDERS

Erin Tolbert, RN, FNP-C

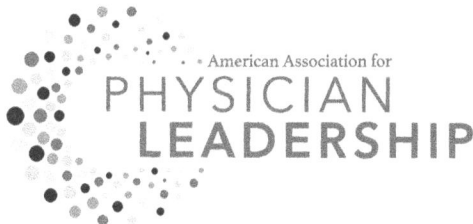

American Association for
PHYSICIAN
LEADERSHIP

PUBLISHER

Nancy Collins

EDITORIAL ASSISTANT

Jennifer Weiss

DESIGN & LAYOUT

Carter Publishing Studio

COPYEDITOR

Pat George

TABLE OF CONTENTS

ACKNOWLEDGMENTS

Writing this book wouldn't have been possible without the support and encouragement of those close to me.

To my husband, Alex Tolbert, I am grateful for your support throughout the process. You encouraged me to take on the project and see it through. Your invaluable insights have helped deepen my knowledge of healthcare, especially in the current political climate, and are apparent throughout this project. I love you the most!

To my publisher, Greenbranch Publishing, thank you for believing in me as I authored this first book, and for the guidance you provided throughout the process. I appreciate your patience with me during the writing process.

To the nurse practitioners and healthcare practices who have shared their stories and experiences with me, I appreciate your transparency and willingness to work together. I am grateful for your partnerships as we navigate the developing world of healthcare and advanced practice professions together.

Finally, to my parents who instilled in me the value of education and of attaining a noble profession, I am eternally grateful. Your influence continues to guide my personal and professional endeavors and has given me a foundation that has taken me further than I ever imagined.

ABOUT THE AUTHOR

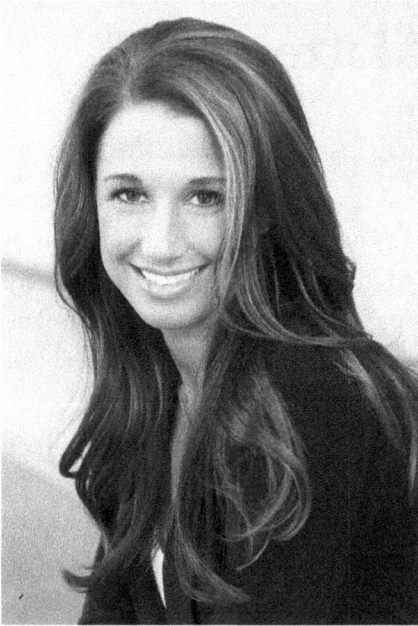

Erin Tolbert is a certified family nurse practitioner who practices in the emergency department in Nashville, Tennessee. She received a Bachelor of Science degree from Vanderbilt University in 2006 with a concentration in molecular and cellular biology and a Master of Science in Nursing degree from Vanderbilt University in 2008. Her clinical experience lies in family practice, urgent care, and emergency medicine.

Based on her own career journey, Erin founded MidlevelU in 2012 to share her professional experience with prospective and practicing nurse practitioners and physician assistants. MidlevelU serves as a resource for NPs, PAs, and the facilities that employ such providers and is a thriving online community with more than 100,000 monthly readers.

Midlevels for the Medically Underserved, the company's residency-like program for nurse practitioners and physician assistants, helps facilitate the transition from education to practice for new providers while serving as a valuable recruitment and retention tool for healthcare facilities in underserved areas nationwide.

Erin and MidlevelU regularly receive national media attention on news outlets like The Fox News Channel and CNN, where Erin appears as a medical expert discussing the latest healthcare news topics.

When she's not working night shift in the emergency department or writing articles for MidlevelU, Erin enjoys running, biking, taking in Nashville's live music scene, traveling to warm-weather destinations, and spending time with her husband and two dogs.

Contact Erin at erin.tolbert@midlevelu.com.

Why Better Midlevel Provider Management Matters

Three short years and three jobs into my nurse practitioner career, I could see them: the cracks in the foundation of our healthcare system. Not only did these problems affect patient care, they reached my personal and professional life as a nurse practitioner. While media drew attention to macro issues, namely healthcare reform, and physicians discussed burnout and dismal reimbursement rates in online forums, little attention was drawn to the advanced practice profession. I knew this needed to change.

In 2012, I founded MidlevelU (midlevelu.com), now a thriving online community of nurse practitioners and physician assistants with over 100,000 monthly visitors. MidlevelU touches on personal, professional, and educational issues and interests advanced practice providers face. Interacting with MidlevelU's growing audience confirmed what I had suspected: I wasn't alone in my career dissatisfaction and fast track to burnout.

Nurse practitioners are educated in a manner much different from that of physicians, then dumped into similar clinical roles. As a new nurse practitioner, this disconnect left me feeling unprepared for my job responsibilities. I had completed my undergraduate education, graduating magna cum laude from Vanderbilt University with a degree in molecular and cellular biology along with a minor in chemistry, a full year ahead of schedule. Aside from one lonely physics course that I was unable to cram into my fast-tracked graduation schedule, I had also tackled all of the required prerequisite courses necessary to apply to medical school. Although I never took the MCAT or applied to medical school, all signs pointed to my promise as a capable clinician.

However, despite my potential for success in the clinical environment, I often felt that my nurse practitioner education, first employers, and system in which I worked were not set up for me to practice to my full potential. Inexperienced and often left to practice on my own, or with the limited help of other busy providers whose productivity suffered should they take the time to offer assistance, I was overwhelmed as a new graduate. In the clinics where I worked, numbers mattered. I was competitive but found it difficult to enhance my clinical knowledge while beating the clock and playing the "billing game."

The MidlevelU community tells me they have experienced similar frustrations. A lack of understanding of the NP and PA education leaves new graduates practicing in environments unsafe for the inexperienced provider. Likewise, physicians and practice managers quickly become frustrated with midlevel providers, deeming them incompetent or not worth the effort to train. Such lack of understanding and contention leads to turnover in advanced practice positions, creating logistical problems for healthcare employers and career dissatisfaction among NPs, PAs, and MDs alike.

On the surface, the natural solution to this problem may seem to be exclusively hiring physicians to join your practice. By doing so, however, medical practices miss out on the benefits midlevel providers can provide. In the face of tight revenue models and the increasing bureaucracy of the healthcare system, our practices are short on time and money. Hiring advanced practice providers offers practices a cost-effective way to increase revenues, offload some of the heavy patient-care burden that leads to physician burnout and, if done well, offers physicians the elusive work-life balance they seek.

To attain such an outcome, physicians and administrators must approach the hiring and management of advanced practice providers with intentionality and understanding. They must implement systems and processes for the recruitment and management of NPs and PAs. Improved management techniques not only to help increase revenues in your practice, but also to create the kind of healthy, thriving practice culture that is lacking in healthcare today.

A NOTE ON THE WORD "MIDLEVEL"

I get a lot of criticism for using the word "midlevel" to describe nurse practitioners and physician assistants. Not one for semantics, I chose to name my company, MidlevelU, based on the current nomenclature in my own workplace at the time. Since then, numerous proposals for naming the collective nurse practitioner and physician assistant professions have surfaced.

Some practices refer to these providers as "physician extenders." The most popular and politically correct title of the times is "advanced practice provider." One nurse practitioner admonished me for not using the term "associate provider." Because the role of these professions is still developing, we can expect to see even more alternate titles in the future.

While some in healthcare consider the term "midlevel provider" to be degrading, I believe it's because they misinterpret the term to mean that NPs and PAs do mediocre work. Instead, I believe the phrase is appropriate for the following reasons:

1. A nurse practitioner functions differently than a nurse. When the nurse practitioner feels uncomfortable handling a complicated patient in a hospital or clinic setting, the NP asks a physician for help or the patient is referred to a physician or another NP with more specialized training. In other words, when it comes to acuity of work, NPs fall in the middle, between the nurse's level and the physician's.
2. I planned to attend medical school to become a physician, but considering the length of time in school and the cost, decided it was not the right path for me. That said, I wanted more autonomy than that of a nurse. So, I chose something in the middle.

When it comes to the quality of care NPs and PAs deliver, I believe they deliver an incredibly high level of care within the scope of care that they have chosen to specialize in, which is that of a nurse practitioner or physician assistant. I do not intend the term "midlevel" to refer to the standard of care NPs deliver.

The purpose of this book is not to engage in a debate about professional nomenclature, but rather to explore the best practices for utilizing nurse practitioners and physician assistants effectively. Throughout this book, I use the terms "midlevel provider" and "advanced practice provider" to refer to nurse practitioners and physician assistants. Whatever your perspective on these phrases, I hope you will not let this detract from the information and guidance this book offers.

Also, please note the names of colleagues have been changed throughout the book to protect their privacy.

Introduction

Many healthcare companies are getting it all wrong when it comes to utilizing nurse practitioners in their clinics and hospitals. Business practices such as productivity-based compensation and bonuses spell death for workplace cultures and doom employment relationships from day one. This is particularly true for new midlevel providers who require help and coaching on *how* to do a good job; factual information from clinical references alone won't teach them.

In many ways, the administrators and physicians who make decisions about the recruitment and role of midlevel providers in these practices are to blame. They may have employed a nurse practitioner or physician assistant in the past who "didn't work out," or "couldn't keep up." So, moving forward, they take steps that they assume will prevent similar problems in the future.

For example, rather than have a difficult conversation with an employee and implement an improvement plan, which requires managerial effort and skill, many practices implement productivity-based compensation as a way to incentivize midlevel providers to take on higher patient volumes and deter those who may be indolent or inefficient from remaining with the practice. The practice may see an initial boost in production and revenue growth with productivity-based compensation, but ultimately such decisions limit a company's ability to grow, and result in long-term decline.

In other cases, practices may have hired a new graduate midlevel provider in the past, not realizing the NP or PA would need continued training in the clinical setting as a new provider. There were no structures to onboard new providers, so the NP or PA failed to meet expectations. The practice vowed never to hire new graduates again, a policy that can result in costly provider vacancies and one that means missing out on midlevel providers who have promising potential—again, limiting the organization's ability to grow.

With simple improvements to the way employment is structured for NPs and PAs, practices can benefit tremendously by using midlevel providers. Midlevel providers can increase revenues, improve practice efficiency, and provide better work-life balance for the provider group as a whole. However, to enjoy these benefits, practices must implement an effective framework for midlevel provider management.

This book examines the common experiences of midlevel providers and explains how you can unlock the potential of midlevel medical providers in your practice. It discusses what you can expect when hiring a midlevel provider and how to help nurse practitioners and physician assistants in your practice reach their full potential. You'll find actionable modifications you can make in your practice to recruit, hire, train, and retain midlevel medical providers in a mutually beneficial employment relationship.

In essence, this is a playbook for using advanced practice providers in such a way that not only are *they* happy and fulfilled, your practice grows and thrives as a result. The key is doing what's best for your practice *and* for your employees.

CHAPTER 1

A Day in the Life of a Midlevel Medical Provider

My own story: pros, cons, and potential to improve

As the end of my nurse practitioner graduate program neared, I kicked off my job search. Having attended an accelerated program designed for students without a background in medicine, I had never worked as a nurse, an EMT, or a medical assistant. My healthcare experience prior to entering school consisted of four months of volunteer work in Kenya and a childhood with an emergency physician father who often told stories at the dinner table that others might deem inappropriate and who commonly escorted his children through the back doors of the hospital for off-the-record X-rays of sports-related injuries.

My resume was appropriately padded with volunteer commitments and summer biology lab internships that required preparing vats of *Drosophila* food, manning a supply of mice and mosquitoes for malaria research, and participating in efforts to sequence the structural proteins of the red blood cell. My science background was robust for someone without real-life professional experience, but my hands-on patient care knowledge was limited to the 750 hours or so of clinical preceptorships I completed as part of my nurse practitioner education.

Despite my anemic healthcare resume, I elicited a response after submitting my CV to several local clinics. My experience at the first and only clinic with which I interviewed in person should have clued me in to the fact that my first job would not be what I was expecting on interpersonal and professional levels.

After making a good impression in my interview with the practice owner, I was invited back for a second interview with the physician who would be supervising me in the clinic. I met the physician at the clinic, and she suggested that I drive us to a nearby restaurant for lunch. (She rode a Harley Davidson motorcycle and could not accommodate a passenger.) So, we climbed into my Jeep, old and rattling but thankfully clean, and drove to the restaurant. Over grilled chicken salads at a generic chain restaurant, she offered me a job. I accepted on the spot.

The practice had three locations scattered across various Nashville, Tennessee, suburbs and catered to walk-in and primary care patients. Each clinic staffed a single physician and several advanced practice providers. My employment agreement in 2008 specified a $40/hour compensation rate as well as a quarterly incentive productivity bonus capping out at nearly $25,000 annually. Motivated, with a strong work ethic and competitive spirit, I assumed I would most certainly maximize the productivity incentive.

I quickly realized my clinical skills had room for improvement. As a new graduate, I lacked procedural training. I had never sutured a laceration or performed an I&D on an abscess, skills essential to the job responsibilities of a nurse practitioner in the walk-in setting. New to prescribing, I constantly had questions about medications, interactions, and dosages. When it came to diagnosing patients, I second-guessed myself and lived in a constant state of uncertainty.

Fortunately, the physician overseeing the clinic where I practiced proved to be an ally. She patiently helped guide me through my inexperience. Then she quit. Unclear expectations, dispute over compensation, and differences in opinion over practice management with the physician owner had her headed for the door. So, there I was, an inexperienced nurse practitioner without a support system.

My nurse practitioner and physician assistant coworkers were helpful but not as effective in training me as my former supervising physician. Somewhat green themselves, they offered clinical advice and judgment that was a bit lacking. And, like me, my midlevel coworkers were also allured by the promise of a productivity bonus. Taking time to assist me meant subtracting from their bottom-line. In a sense, we were competing with each other for patients when we would have been more effective as a collaborative group.

To further complicate matters, the practice had implemented measures to increase revenues in an increasingly strapped healthcare landscape—most notably the offering of certain diagnostic testing services. NPs and PAs, for example, were encouraged to order echocardiograms liberally, a service offered on site at the clinic every Friday. Young, low-risk patients, without indications for doing so, often received such testing. Tympanometry testing was another revenue-generating test offered on site that was encouraged. Such tests increased practice revenues, the reality of which I was made acutely aware by administrators.

My disenchantment with the practice was heightened by the fact that test results were interpreted by a physician family member of the practice owner, an incestuous referral pool that raised red flags from my perspective. Furthermore, midlevel providers were not provided training or resources regarding the clinical necessity of such tests. Articles outlining clinical guidelines for use of these diagnostic tools never hit our inboxes. This left us with the feeling that very few of the tests we ordered in-house were relevant.

Profits were the primary goal of the practice, setting the tone for the negative practice culture. Midlevel providers were encouraged to function in a manner that maximized revenue rather than one centered around clinical guidelines.

To some degree, my negative experience can be chalked up to the disillusionment that many healthcare providers experience in their first years of practice. The realization that medicine is a business and that one's aspirations to "help people" often take a back seat is a common frustration among healthcare providers. The reality is, practices must keep themselves afloat financially; however, subjecting patients to unnecessary testing in order to bill insurance carriers, caused me to lose respect for my employer.

My compensation structure placed me in a position of moral compromise. Should I order diagnostic tests offered by the practice to maximize my productivity bonus all the while knowing the result of the test was unhelpful? Or, should I omit unnecessary testing from my diagnosis and treatment plan at the expense of my paycheck?

A similar revenue-generating scenario proved even more compromising, as it potentially endangered patients or at least led to substandard patient care. The clinic housed an X-ray machine, and ordering X-rays on site rather than at the outpatient radiology center next door was naturally encouraged.

The availability of on-site X-rays was convenient for both patients and providers. Billing for such basic diagnostic testing did not seem excessive; the convenience of X-ray capabilities at a walk-in clinic was obvious. The problem was that midlevel providers were encouraged to not send X-rays out for interpretation by a radiologist, as the cost of interpretation cut into clinic profits.

The less-experienced midlevel providers did not feel comfortable interpreting many X-rays taken in the clinic. Coaching and training on X-ray interpretation could have remedied this disconnect, yet none was offered. We were left on our own to interpret X-rays with inadequate training at the expense of providing safe patient care. Pressure to increase profits and earn productivity incentives left midlevel providers and the practice exposed to legal liability.

This tension created by billing pressures created dissatisfaction among midlevel providers in the clinic. We often felt like used car salesmen, convincing patients they might benefit from an echocardiogram all the while knowing the test was likely unnecessary and that we would personally take a cut of the bill. Needless to say, provider turnover in the practice was high.

With the end of the calendar year came time to dole out bonuses. Despite working in a busy clinic with a chronically packed waiting room, none of the NPs or PAs, including me, received bonuses that year. It was then that I realized I had been careless in signing my employment agreement. The incentive structure was nebulous and not clearly delineated in my contract. Whether I deserved a bonus that year or not, without a clearly outlined bonus compensation structure to point to, I will never know. I ate my perceived losses and instantly lost trust with my employer. My NP and PA coworkers shared my sentiments.

Bitterness over bonuses and mistrust over the owner's pressure to increase revenues through ancillary services were eating away at the practice. Turnover among staff, and particularly among midlevel providers was high. Negative attitudes poisoned the clinic culture, leaving staff and providers aligned in their distaste for the company and their jobs in general. Nearly all of this dissent among NPs and PAs stemmed from a lack of support, billing pressures and the way midlevel providers' compensation was structured.

After a nearly 12-month term, true to the practice's turnover trend, I handed in my resignation. My boss threatened to sue me if left, stating that I was in breach of contract, leaving my position before my one-year employment anniversary had officially arrived. He also tossed other legal allegations such as "patient abandonment" into our conversation. I became even more bitter about my experience.

Looking back, I must have been more productive than my nonexistent bonus indicated, given his misguided attempt to keep me. I signed on with a local urgent care clinic an easy five-minute commute from my home that also came with a $5 an hour increase in pay.

THE DISCONNECT—WHY HEALTHCARE PROVIDERS ENTER THE MEDICAL FIELD

Medical providers—nurse practitioners, physician assistants, and physicians alike—enter the medical field for one of two reasons:

1. To earn a good living in a stable profession; or
2. To have a career centered around helping others.

Unfortunately, despite what would seem like solid reasoning, these providers often find themselves dissatisfied.

Earning a living as a motivation for a healthcare career = dissatisfaction.

I enrolled in Vanderbilt University in 2003, an institution packed with premed students like me. I majored in molecular and cellular biology with a minor in chemistry. Intent on a career as a physician, I fast-tracked my education with the goal of graduating in just three years. Most of my classmates, including me, did not enter premed studies based on a passion for patient care. Rather, we were identified as students with an interest in or talent for the sciences, so a career in medicine seemed like a natural fit. Working in a biochemistry lab is less likely to pay a six-figure salary than working in healthcare, so students gravitated to medicine as a career path catering to a passion for science, the human body, and a substantial paycheck.

There is nothing inherently wrong with entering a profession for financial gain. However, students are idealistic when it comes to salaries for healthcare providers. Naive to the ever-growing healthcare bureaucracy and the logistics of working with third-party payers, their visions of financial grandeur are quickly squashed when real life sets in.

As healthcare providers, we quickly become disillusioned, feeling that our compensation is threatened by government whims and practice mismanagement. Provider salaries are under constant threat as reimbursement rates are challenged and the face of healthcare changes. Even highly specialized physicians with top salaries experience the anxiety of such changes, contributing to career dissatisfaction and burnout.

Helping people as a motivation for a healthcare career = dissatisfaction.

Most of us aren't entirely altruistic in selecting our career paths, but the allure of "doing good" and "making a difference" is attractive. We may have watched a friend or family member struggle through an illness and want to support families in similar situations. We may have volunteered in an impoverished community, witnessing the failed state of healthcare, and plan to use our education to make a difference for underserved patient populations. Whatever prompts our motivation to "help," in practice, our good intentions become clouded by the way our facilities operate and by government and insurance company red tape.

Primary care in particular suffers from these realities. Prospective healthcare providers entering the field with a benevolent mindset often envision themselves interacting with patients similar to the stereotypical family doctors of the past, caring for patients from birth to death. However, compensation for such providers is low compared to that of those in specialties. The burden of government red tape hits already-strapped primary care providers the hardest. As a result, providers who entered the medical field to make a difference in patients' lives find their career objectives unattainable and are reduced to working in jobs that don't match up with their professional passions.

This disconnect is particularly hard on nurse practitioners. Nurse practitioners are unique among healthcare providers in that they typically have a background in nursing. Some NPs enter the field with many years of experience working on the hospital floor. As nurses, they have witnessed the effects of unmanaged chronic disease on patients. They have wiped the rear ends of patients suffering with C. diff as the result of inappropriately prescribed antibiotics. So, they advance their education with the intention of stopping the cycle of acute and chronic illness before it starts.

Quickly, new NPs realize that despite their good intentions, health coaching doesn't pay. Visions of changing patients' eating habits to prevent diabetes and encouraging exercise to combat hypertension vanish. Such conversations are not "productive" from a practice's perspective—at least not to the extent that is typically required to facilitate a change in behavior. Reimbursement rates for office visits are low, so NPs are encouraged to pack a greater number of patients into their schedules, leaving little time for health coaching. Procedures and diagnostic tests pay, and are more likely to be encouraged by practice management than conversation. Working with a constant awareness of compensation is inevitable and draining.

HEALTHCARE PROVIDERS AS SALESPEOPLE

Reimbursement based on the fee-for-service model has essentially turned healthcare providers into commissioned salespeople. Our paychecks depend on ordering diagnostic testing, performing procedures, and fitting more patients into our schedules. Our "commissions" are paid by third parties that dictate how we must practice. The more time we spend with our patients, the less we earn. The more quickly we can "sell" a few diagnostic tests and churn patients in and out of our facilities, however, the more satisfied our employers and the fatter our wallets. This type of model is soul-crushing for those who entered the profession with the intention of helping others.

Unlike sales in most industries, however, healthcare providers "sell" to a population with limited ability to purchase other products or use other services. Bills are ultimately paid by the government or insurance companies so the effect of being "sold to" has a limited impact on the patients' own finances.

The current healthcare infrastructure also restricts where patients may turn for healthcare needs. Insurance carriers, for example, may cover one facility and not another. The result is interrupted competition among medical providers and healthcare facilities, hampering the motivation to excel in providing patient care. When patients are told where they must go for care, there's no need to stand out among competing facilities. This reality, coupled with incentives to tailor care in a manner that maximizes revenues as dictated by the government and insurance companies, results in dissatisfaction among healthcare providers and discourages quality patient care.

Inevitably, even providers with integrity will be influenced by commissions as part of fee-for-service compensation structures. Practicing with a constant awareness of how each clinical intervention affects one's paycheck influences how a provider practices. Research shows a direct link between provider compensation and the manner in which medical care is provided.

In one study, for example, a major chain of ambulatory care centers replaced hourly wages with bonuses determined by revenue generated. The number of laboratory tests performed per patient visit increased by 23% and the number of X-rays ordered increased by 16% in conjunction with the change.[1] Tying compensation directly to productivity prompts providers to sell more services.

While such compensation models may provide an initial bump in revenue, ultimately the structure of our healthcare system places healthcare providers in a morally compromising situation. It rewards actions rather than results. Misaligned incentives result in guilt, resentment, frustration, and burnout. Dissatisfaction even hits providers who entered the profession without magnanimous intentions.

As healthcare providers, we may hope to find value in our profession based on the fact that we are compassionate, personable, helpful, knowledgeable, or excel in the clinical sense. We do not enter the medical field looking for a career pitching our services. But, that is what our health system has made us. We pitch diagnostic tests and other services patients may or may not need to earn a few extra dollars. The system is not structured to effectively help patients. This disparity leads to job dissatisfaction, turnover, and negative work environments.

The fee-for-service reimbursement model creates a natural framework for employers to structure provider compensation on a productivity rather than a salaried basis. Employers operate under the assumption that productivity-based compensation rewards highly productive providers and weeds out those less motivated. Compensation directly tied to one's day-to-day performance is implemented as a motivational tool. Productivity-based compensation models, however, reinforce the faults in the structure of our healthcare system.

While productivity-based incentives may seem to influence providers to work in a way that positively affects revenues, the compensation model is ultimately a detriment to medical practices. Productivity compensation structures are complex and often misunderstood by providers. This sets the stage for mistrust between the employer and employee. It encourages competition rather than teamwork among coworkers, resulting in a negative practice culture. The concept of healthcare providers as salespeople, and the moral conflict created by productivity-based pay, is reinforced in the practice itself, leading to frustration, burnout, and turnover among staff.

PRACTICE MISMANAGEMENT WOES

In 2010, following my year-long stint in the walk-in/primary care setting, I joined a local urgent care clinic chain and received a small bump in pay to $45/hour. As an added perk, the clinic where I was assigned was located a mere two miles from my home. The arrangement seemed promising and free of the compensation frustrations I experienced in my prior position.

The urgent care clinic compensated nurse practitioners on a flat hourly basis, the simplicity of which was attractive to me. Efficiency was encouraged, however excessive billing pressures were distant. Unlike at my previous job, a physician was present to assist with my developing X-ray interpretation skills and procedural abilities. Midlevel providers' skills were accurately perceived based on level of experience, and physicians showed an interest in helping NPs and PAs reach their full potential.

While billing pressures were minimized by the hourly compensation model, at least for midlevel providers, practice mismanagement was rife. Unlike midlevel providers, physicians in the urgent care clinic were compensated on a productivity basis. To keep up with patient volume, each MD had the option of requesting a midlevel provider to help out. The midlevel provider's wages, or at least a portion of them, were then deducted from the physician's paycheck.

Although this appeared fair, as it rewarded efficient, highly productive physicians, it subjected midlevel providers to unpredictable staffing whims. When the clinic was slow, midlevel providers were sent home so the physician could avoid paying for unneeded help from his or her own wallet. If a physician decided during a slow season that he or she no longer wanted help, the midlevel provider would lose his or her job or be shuffled around to help cover occupational health contracts held by the company. I was the subject of the latter such transition.

I adored the physician I worked with. She was experienced and an excellent mentor. We had a solid working relationship built on mutual trust and respect. When volume at the urgent care clinic dropped for a period of time, however, she opted to work solo, without midlevel provider assistance. I understood her position and could not blame her decision despite my disappointment. I was reassigned to cover an employee health clinic more than an hour away from my home.

The clinic I was assigned to serviced a large number of primary care and occupational health patients, a specialty I was trying to distance myself from. The commute also began to wear on me. Practice mismanagement and unclear expectations left me dissatisfied. Other providers experienced similar problems and the workplace culture quickly took a turn for the worse.

I quickly began to hate my job. I often purchased Powerball tickets at the gas station on my way home from work in hopes I would win the jackpot and be able to quit. My luck with the lottery dismal, I started back on the job interview circuit, this time targeting my ultimate goal of securing employment in the emergency department.

THE ROOT OF MISMANAGEMENT

Physicians receive notoriously little, if any, business training in medical school. However, they find themselves working in managerial roles. Both solo physicians and those working for large hospital systems must act like business owners. They make decisions regarding management, recruitment, and retention of employees. They are responsible for delegating, motivating, and empowering those who work for and alongside them. These responsibilities are required in conjunction with providing patient care services.

Not only are physicians charged with patient care, they must also keep up with the new advancements in medicine in order to provide evidence-based care. Who has time to read management books as well as medical journals? Who can devote time to managerial training while also keeping up with the government's latest healthcare delivery mandates or learning to use a new EHR system? Without basic management training and adequate time to devote to administrative tasks, physicians often find themselves ineffective in these roles.

Effective management is especially necessary in healthcare. Most of the problems our healthcare system faces are related to business and politics, not patient care. The complexities of the healthcare system present a challenge to even the most capable corporate CEO, let alone a solo physician without any managerial training. Success balancing the responsibilities of maintaining one's own patient panel along with the responsibilities associated with operating a business is rare.

A number of practice woes follow mismanagement. Physicians themselves become frustrated and burn out without the skills, energy, or desire to address managerial issues the practice faces. The result is employee turnover. The remaining staff must assume additional responsibilities, and the cycle of turnover continues as employees, frustrated by the increased workload and resulting disorganization, elect to move on as well. A negative workplace culture takes root, affecting productivity and revenues. Recruiting and hiring new staff is costly and time consuming. The mismanagement cycle is difficult to break, particularly without a background in business management.

COMPENSATION STRUCTURES AND COMPETITION

Frustrated with the workplace culture and management at the urgent care clinic where I worked, I began exploring employment in an emergency department. Through a professional connection, I landed an interview at a local hospital for an emergency department nurse practitioner opening and was offered the job at the end of my interview.

Overall, the emergency department was managed much more competently than my previous places of employment. The physicians with whom I worked put effort into my training, helping me become an asset to the team of providers. Still, as in my first job, underlying pressure to bill and compensation structured around productivity left their mark on the work environment.

In the emergency department, physicians were compensated entirely based on productivity. Midlevel providers earned a base salary that was supplemented by additional RVU-based compensation. On average, my paycheck amounted to about 50% hourly base pay and 50% RVU-based compensation.

The productivity-based compensation structure often led to an underlying competitive vibe in the department and undermined our ability to work together more efficiently. When I was called in to assist a physician with a procedure rather than see a patient of my own, for example, I was sacrificing pay. Patients with chief complaints known to reimburse at lower rates would linger in the to-be-seen chart rack while charts for patients with problems with high reimbursement rates were snatched up immediately. Comments like "this fracture is going to pay for my kid's new shoes" were common, demonstrating the constant awareness of compensation.

The intention of productivity-based compensation was to reward highly motivated, competent providers; however, it was detrimental to overall workplace efficiency and cooperation. It limited our ability to explore methods for staffing the department more effectively. Again, the compensation model was accompanied with the misaligned incentive that ordering more tests and procedures directly affected our wallets. Ultimately, the structure of my compensation was not conducive to providing the best value and care to my patients, at times placing me in a morally compromising situation.

IN SUMMARY

Overall, the methods by which employers compensate, train, and prepare midlevel medical providers does not take full advantage of their strengths. Instead, midlevel providers are treated like salespeople, mismanaged, or both. High turnover, burnout, and improper use of both providers' and employers' time are the results. Ultimately, these factors impact revenues and patient care.

Fortunately, there is a real opportunity to improve a practice's revenues by leveraging midlevel providers' strengths. Midlevel salaries are lower than those of physicians and they can be used to free-up physician's time for more interesting and complex cases or improved work-life balance. With appropriate mentoring, training and management, midlevel providers can be a valued ally for physicians and one that sticks around for the long haul.

REFERENCE

1. Kingma, M. Can financial incentive influence medical practice? *Human Resources for Health Development Journal*, 1999, 3(2):121–131.

CHAPTER 2

A Look Inside How Providers Are Educated

Understanding where midlevel providers come from and how they got there

I spoke recently with a physician medical director for a major health system in the Chicago area. Our conversation centered around the system's nurse practitioner staffing strategy. "Our physicians just aren't quite sure what to do with NPs," he lamented. Recognizing the value proposition that utilizing midlevel providers offers, the hospital had opted to hire NPs and PAs in conjunction with additional physicians to accommodate increasing patient volume. The experiment was not going well.

"Some of our docs treat nurse practitioners like medical residents," the medical director explained. The expectation that NPs work an excess number of hours compared with the terms that had been outlined in the hiring process wasn't welcomed by the new midlevel provider team.

"Other physicians delegate very little responsibility to midlevel providers," he said. "They aren't using them effectively, and have little clarity as to their role."

While state scope of practice laws makes hiring midlevel providers trickier in Illinois than in some other states, the way in which the midlevel providers were onboarded by practice administration and the treatment of them by physicians was defeating the purpose of the hospital's plan. High turnover among those in departments where nurse practitioners were treated like medical residents proved costly. Underutilization of advanced practice providers in other departments undermined the clinical and financial value of employing nurse practitioners and physician assistants.

Nurse practitioners, physician assistants, and physicians are all different as professionals. Their education, skill sets, and scope of practice are unique. Without knowledge as to how midlevel providers are trained, the benefits of using midlevel medical providers may be lost. Understanding the educational path of advanced practice providers as well as the realities of what it takes to integrate them into the practice environment is essential to a successful working relationship.

HOW NURSE PRACTITIONERS ARE EDUCATED

There are several paths by which nurse practitioners are educated. Most follow one of three pathways:

1. Traditional approach;
2. Stepwise approach; or
3. Direct entry approach.

Each of these approaches leads to the same end: becoming a certified nurse practitioner. These approaches must be taken into account in hiring and training decisions as they affect the level of experience of the individual NP.

Traditional approach

The most common path to the nurse practitioner profession is to obtain a four-year bachelor's degree in nursing (BSN) followed by a master's degree in nursing (MSN), or a doctorate of nursing practice (DNP). Typically, a master's degree takes from one to three years to complete; a doctorate degree takes two to four years to complete. Most nurses are employed in the healthcare setting for a number of months to years before returning to school for a master's or doctorate degree, although nursing experience is not required for acceptance to many NP programs.

Stepwise approach

Another route aspiring nurse practitioners may take to enter practice is a more lengthy, stepwise approach. Students on this path first obtain an RN degree from an associate's level program. They may then opt to complete a bachelor's degree in nursing (BSN) or apply directly to a nurse practitioner program specifically modeled for students with an associate's level degree. Like NPs entering the profession in a traditional manner, nurse practitioners beginning their career as associate's level nurses typically have nursing experience before becoming NPs.

Direct entry approach

Select schools such as Columbia University, Yale University, and Vanderbilt University offer accelerated pathways for students with a bachelor's degree in a field other than nursing to become nurse practitioners. These programs go by a variety of titles, including accelerated programs, bridge programs, or master's entry programs in nursing (MEPN). Schools offering such fast-tracked programs award both nursing and nurse practitioner degrees in just two to three years, attended on a full-time basis. The first year of the program, students learn basic nursing skills, earning an RN degree. The second year of the program, students complete coursework and clinical hours required to earn an MSN degree, allowing them to become nurse practitioners.

Direct entry programs typically attract students looking to nursing as a second profession, along with those who did not focus on nursing early in their undergraduate education. While these graduates lack healthcare experience, having not previously worked as nurses, they may have other professional experience and maturity that outweigh the absence of a background in nursing.

This is the type of program I completed on my own path to becoming an NP. Unaware that the nurse practitioner profession was an option early in my undergraduate years, I had nearly completed my bachelor's degree before I decided on my profession. So, after completing my undergraduate education, I enrolled in Vanderbilt University's two-year accelerated program, earning my RN degree in one year and my MSN as a family nurse practitioner in the second year of the program.

The Doctorate of Nursing Practice (DNP)

Recent lobbying efforts by national nursing organizations have called for the requirement of a doctorate-level degree for nurse practitioners. In 2004, the American Association of Colleges of Nursing (AACN) published a statement recommending that by 2015, nurse practitioner programs and state governments require the DNP rather than the MSN for entry into nurse practitioner practice.

The requested doctoral mandate intended to further nurse practitioner education on a practical, practice-based level rather than focus on research like the PhD. Advocates of the mandate argue that the DNP is necessary to establish rapport of nurse practitioners on a level similar to other health professions. Audiologists, pharmacists, and physical therapists, for example, may hold doctorate degrees. Opponents argue that requiring a doctorate serves only to lengthen NP education and increase its cost. DNP programs require students to complete very few, if any, clinical hours in a hands-on practice setting similar to medical residencies. Rather, curriculum centers around completion of a capstone project that investigates a practice-based problem. The DNP is not currently a requirement for entry to nurse practitioner practice, but is increasing in popularity.

HOW PHYSICIAN ASSISTANTS ARE EDUCATED

Like the nurse practitioner profession, there are multiple paths for the completion of the physician assistant education. They can be categorized as follows:
1. Traditional approach; and
2. Accelerated approach

Traditional approach

The majority of physician assistants begin their education by obtaining a bachelor's degree. Then, following an undergraduate education, enroll in a master's level physician assistant program that is completed in about 24 to 28 months.

Within this traditional approach to the PA education, schools can be divided into two main categories: those that require applicants to have healthcare experience and those that do not. Most physician assistant programs require anywhere from a few hundred to a few thousand hours of direct patient care experience as a prerequisite for admission. So, these programs attract individuals previously employed in the healthcare sector such as EMTs and medical assistants.

A handful of schools do not require that physician assistant program applicants have a background in healthcare. While experience in healthcare may not be a prerequisite for admission, these schools still strongly encourage such experience and consider this as part of a competitive application package. Still, it is possible to become a physician assistant without a healthcare background.

Accelerated approach

As with nurse practitioners, a small number of colleges and universities offer a fast-track to the PA profession. Students without a four-year bachelor's degree, or who are embarking on their undergraduate education, may enroll in a BS/MS program that shaves about one year off the traditional education path for physician assistants. These programs award a bachelor's degree, typically in life sciences, as well as a master of science in physician assistant studies upon graduation. Overall, these programs take about five years to complete.

EDUCATION COMPARISON

Both physician assistant and nurse practitioner programs consist of didactic and clinical education. The number of clinical hours completed in each program depends on the provider's specialty and the college or university itself. Table 2.1 compares the average length of education of nurse practitioners, physician assistants, and physicians.

TABLE 2.1. Length of Education: NP vs. PA vs. MD

	Undergraduate	Graduate	Residency	Total Time
Nurse Practitioner (MSN, DNP)	4-year BA or BS	1 to 4-year master's or doctoral program	None required	5 to 8 years
Physician Assistant (MPAS)	4-year BA or BS	2 to 2 1/2-year master's program	None required	6 to 6 1/2 years
Physician (D.O., MD)	4-year BA or BS	4-year medical program	Minimum 3-year requirement	Minimum 11 years

Length of training is not the only component that factors into scope of practice and proficiency of members of each profession in the clinical setting. The number of hours spent training in the direct patient care setting translates into the experience most relevant to the employment. Table 2.2 compares the estimated number of clinical hours completed as part of the nurse practitioner, physician assistant, and physician education.

Overall, physicians spend significantly more time on their overall education than NPs and PAs. This includes the approximately 10 times more hours in the clinical setting.

TABLE 2.2. Clinical Hours Required in Education: NP vs. PA vs. MD

	Clinical Hours in Program	Residency Hours	Total Clinical Hours
Nurse Practitioner (MSN, DNP)	500 to 1,500	None required	500 to 1,500
Physician Assistant (MPAS)	2,000	None required	2,000
Physician (D.O., MD)	6,000	9,000 to 10,000	15,000 to 16,000

While midlevel providers and physicians have very different educational backgrounds, this isn't always taken into account in staffing, hiring, and managerial decisions. Neglecting to understand these educational realities leads to frustration on the part of both advanced practice providers and employers, setting the relationship up for failure.

A NOTE ON ONLINE EDUCATION

In my conversations with employers related to nurse practitioners and physician assistants, many express concerns about hiring providers with online education. As I describe my company's residency-like program for NPs and PAs, hospitals and clinics are on board with the concept, but skeptically ask "What schools do your applicants come from? Are these NPs from online schools?" Doubts about the merits of online education for healthcare providers are common and understandable given that patient care requires a hands-on skill set.

Online Education for Nurse Practitioners

Online programs for nurse practitioners are prevalent. These schools teach didactic course content remotely, in a live or recorded forum. In addition to viewing lecture content, coursework may include participation in online discussion boards rather than via face-to-face interactions. Hands-on clinical education is completed via a series of rotations in the live clinical setting at a facility convenient to the nurse practitioner. In some cases, schools arrange clinical rotations on students' behalf. In other cases, NP students are responsible for reaching out to healthcare facilities on their own to arrange these rotations.

One downfall of NP education is that it depends heavily on the strength of these clinical rotations. Nurse practitioner students who are unable to identify healthcare providers that are capable teachers and mentors simply do not gain as much valuable experience in their clinical rotations as those paired with stronger instructors. While this is the reality for NPs who attend bricks and mortar schools as well as for those in online programs, I do see that online nurse practitioner students struggle the most with identifying quality clinical rotations.

NPs living in areas with limited access to education and healthcare are more likely to complete online programs than those located nearby these resources. While online programs allow nurse practitioner students in all geographic areas access to education, when it comes to clinical rotations, online students have limited options for mentorship and clinical experience where they are located. Online programs are also less likely to have local resources for students spread across multiple states than locally based schools. In turn, these programs are not as capable of assisting when a student is unable to find a healthcare provider interested in helping with the clinical training component of their program.

Online Education for Physician Assistants

Physician assistant schools have been slow to adopt the online training model. However, as the number of practicing nurse practitioners increases more quickly than the number of practicing physician assistants, the profession is looking at online education as a way to make PA education more readily accessible to aspiring healthcare providers. The Yale School of Medicine is slated to offer the first online physician assistant program and will matriculate its first cohort of students in January 2018.

Based on this inaugural program, online education for physician assistants will look similar to that for nurse practitioners. Foundational didactic coursework may be completed remotely while in-person clinical rotation requirements are fulfilled at various healthcare facilities located as conveniently as possible to the student's home.

DISPARITIES BETWEEN EDUCATION AND REALITY

Studies show that midlevel providers can manage 80% to 90% of the care provided by primary care physicians.[1] However, looking at the length of didactic education and number of clinical hours completed by each type of healthcare provider, this seems like an unrealistic statistic. Can nurse practitioners, whose education may include just 5% of the clinical hours of that of a physician, really function in an analogous role? Of course not. Not initially, at least.

Recently, my company launched Midlevels for the Medically Underserved. The program serves two purposes. First, it helps clinics and hospitals working with underserved populations attract motivated and energetic nurse practitioners and physician assistants to their practices. Second, the program serves as a year of transition from education to practice for participating NPs and PAs. Somewhat analogous to a residency for midlevel providers, NPs and PAs are paired with practices that offer a supportive setting for recent graduates.

As we launched the program, I was surprised by the number of applications we received from experienced nurse practitioners. Why would NPs with experience under their belt voluntarily take the pay cut associated with participating in a residency-like program? As I spoke to these nurse practitioners, a common thread appeared.

An employment history that provided little clinical support left these NPs lacking competency and confidence in their roles as providers. Employers did not provide the resources required to overcome the clinical learning curve they faced. Mismanaged practices expected these nurse practitioners to perform at a higher standard than their level of experience allowed. Patients with complex medical conditions were not triaged to more experienced providers. Rather, new NPs were expected to see complex patients autonomously, without a more experienced clinician available when questions arose.

The learning curve midlevel providers face after graduation is steep. The clinical component required by nurse practitioner and physician assistant programs is not sufficient for these providers to achieve a scope of practice or productivity similar to that of physicians right out of school. So, employers must step in. If they do not, the result is disappointment and frustration on part of both the employer and advanced practice provider.

WHY HIRE INEXPERIENCED MIDLEVEL PROVIDERS?

Given the challenges new midlevel providers face, the natural solution for employers looking to tap into the value advanced practice providers offer is to hire experienced NPs and PAs. In some practice settings, and for some clinics and hospitals, seeking out experienced midlevel providers is the appropriate approach. Practices that treat high-acuity patients, for example, may be best paired with a midlevel provider who has a strong clinical background. Settings where midlevel providers are required to practice alone, with minimal or no backup from other providers, also may rightly shy away from hiring less-experienced NPs and PAs.

On the other hand, some clinics may not have the option to hire experienced midlevel providers, forcing them to look to less-experienced NPs and PAs as a staffing solution. Others would do well to consider less-experienced midlevel providers, recognizing that these NPs and PAs have a lot to offer.

While training a new provider may seem daunting, less-experienced midlevel providers are enthusiastic. They are eager to learn and contribute. They are open to suggestions and feedback. New graduates don't have bad practice habits to break. New NPs and PAs understand the need for continued education to perform to their full potential. Employers can help them reach this goal in a manner that benefits their practice, not to mention, employing new NPs and PAs is a cost-effective staffing measure.

Another benefit of hiring less-experienced midlevel providers is their eagerness to prove themselves in a new career. Energy and a positive attitude can overcome the inconvenience of supporting a new graduate through the transition from education to proficient clinical practice. Less-experienced NPs and PAs may be willing to take on tasks others may not, or to pick up less-than-ideal shifts to gain experience. While healthcare providers who have been in practice for many years often burn out, those with less experience are able to put more energy toward building their career. Their efforts ultimately translate to high levels of productivity and loyalty.

Gary, the Chief Medical Officer of an eight-clinic community health system in southern California, understands this concept and has used it to his advantage in staffing their facilities. "Our support system is busy," he acknowledges. The time to effectively train NPs and PAs can be difficult for physicians and other experienced providers to find. While the company does make an effort to provide structured clinical support for inexperienced providers, they also look for specific qualities in new midlevel providers that have proven effective for success.

"Nurse practitioners and physician assistants who are willing to put in the hours and effort required to excel in their first year of practice end up being very successful," he notes. Gary is up-front with midlevel providers in the hiring process about the learning curve they can expect to face. "They must be willing to take charting and paperwork home after hours, consult resources, and have a solid work ethic," he explains. "Look for the right person, someone willing to put in the effort" when it comes to inexperienced midlevel providers, he advises. Although inexperienced providers do face challenges out of school, the right provider will overcome this learning curve and become an asset to your organization.

THE LEARNING CURVE FOR EXPERIENCED MIDLEVEL PROVIDERS

Hiring experienced nurse practitioners and physician assistants is not a fool-proof tactic for tapping into the value they offer without training and effective management. As discussed earlier, midlevel providers receive some hands-on clinical education as part of their schooling, however they still have a significant amount to learn in the workplace once they graduate. Any gaps in clinical knowledge left by a previous employer, intentionally or otherwise, will still exist when the provider comes on board in your practice.

Hiring a midlevel provider with experience analogous to your practice seems like a slam dunk. Clinical experience translates directly to the patient population at hand, making for a natural transition—or so it seems. In reality, however, hiring a midlevel provider with experience in a given specialty looks very different, depending on the individual provider. One provider may have had excellent support and training early in his or her career while another may not. Years of experience typically help overcome clinical deficits, however areas of clinical weakness may still be present even with experience. You must be prepared to take the time to help the new provider overcome areas of weakness.

State scope of practice laws also must be considered in advanced practice provider hiring decisions. In some states, nurse practitioners and physician assistants have unrestricted ability to diagnose, treat, and prescribe. In others, midlevel providers find their scope of practice significantly limited by state legislation. Hiring a midlevel provider from another state where scope of practice is limited, for a position in a state allowing a higher degree of autonomy, may mean the provider has not had the opportunity to train in certain aspects of practice. Additional instruction will be required.

Decoding Experience

Employers must be cautious in assuming that hiring an NP or PA with experience means that support and training will not be necessary. Such assumptions set the employment relationship up for failure.

To avoid such a misstep, during the interview process, ask midlevel providers to describe their previous role(s). How were they used in the clinic or hospital setting? What responsibilities did they have? How much oversight was provided by physicians and/

or more experienced midlevel providers? This will clue you in as to where you need to focus training efforts should you bring the provider onto your team.

Additionally, ask the provider about areas of clinical weakness. Present the question by letting the provider know you are interested in knowing where to focus training should he or she be offered the position. Providers will appreciate the acknowledgment that clinical training will be necessary and look forward to the challenge of continued learning. Initiating a conversation about clinical weaknesses sets you apart from other employers, indicating to the provider that your facility offers a supportive work environment.

IN SUMMARY

The CMO of a community clinic system in Kansas I spoke with described the new graduate nurse practitioners and physician assistants she hires as "different shades of green." Based on the healthcare background and quality of each individual provider's education, she notices a significant difference in performance. This is the reality of working with NPs and PAs. While midlevel providers offer significant benefits to your organization, their level of education must be taken into account when structuring onboarding, mentorship and setting expectations for performance. Overcoming these educational disparities begins with effective management, which I will discuss in Chapter 4.

REFERENCE

1. Van Vleet A and Paradise J. Tapping nurse practitioners to meet rising demand for primary care. The Henry J. Kaiser Family Foundation. January 20, 2015. http://kff.org/medicaid/issue-brief/tapping-nurse-practitioners-to-meet-rising-demand-for-primary-care. Accessed November 13, 2016.

CHAPTER 3

Educational Differences Among Providers—Call for Effective Management

Setting the tone for midlevel providers with leadership

Given the education disparities between midlevel providers and physicians, effective management of healthcare practices is of utmost importance. Without it, midlevel providers' ability to add value to your business suffers. Too many practices neglect the business and management element associated with hiring NPs, and productivity plummets as a result.

OVERCOMING EDUCATION DISPARITIES WITH EFFECTIVE MANAGEMENT

I hold a clinical position as a nurse practitioner in three emergency departments. While owned by the same healthcare system, each hospital operates quite differently, particularly with respect to employment of midlevel providers. In turn, each gets very different results from NPs and PAs, with the productivity of midlevel providers linked directly back to management practices.

One of my hospital employers offers superior support to the midlevel team. Each physician is assigned a four-hour block of time each shift during which they are responsible for NP and PA oversight in addition to patient care. Midlevel providers' charts are cosigned by the designated physician and any questions the NP or PA has regarding patient care are directed toward this physician during the specified timeframe.

The predicable structure this arrangement provides allows physicians time when they exclusively are responsible for their own patients and evenly distributes the responsibility of assisting less-experienced midlevel providers with higher-acuity patients. The arrangement ensures quality patient care on the part of NPs and PAs, as well as job satisfaction based on the support they receive. A predictable oversight schedule allows each physician to manage his or her time effectively throughout each shift. Ultimately, the oversight arrangement allows the department to handle high patient volumes efficiently, effectively, and safely, as indicated by higher scores on efficiency metrics compared with other area hospitals.

Given this structured system of physician oversight, the emergency department also has the capacity to support newer NP and PA graduates. The department certainly evaluates experience as part of the hiring process, but also looks at motivation and work ethic to a greater extent than do many area employers. New graduates who are a good cultural fit for the team can thrive in the supportive work environment. A system of support allows for hiring decisions based on personality characteristics rather than strictly on clinical ability, creating cohesiveness among the provider team as a whole. Turnover is low. New graduates and midlevel providers with little emergency department experience improve quickly in their clinical skills, requiring less and less support as they grow. The department has few challenges related to provider staffing, and a highly motivated, stable team.

The second emergency department where I work struggles with the education disparity between physicians and midlevel providers. Turnover among midlevel medical providers is high, and taking advantage of the large supply of new graduates coming from area nurse practitioner schools isn't an option. The structure of the department does not allow for training new graduates and getting their clinical skills up to speed.

At this hospital, the charts of patients treated by midlevel providers must be cosigned by a physician based on hospital policy. The department has minimal structure, if any, for delegating the responsibility of cosigning charts. Although most midlevel providers in the department are experienced in the emergency setting, when a question arises, there is no system outlining which physician is responsible for providing assistance. As a result, providers who are seen as the "nicest" and most receptive to requests end up taking on the additional responsibility of overseeing midlevel providers.

A problem arises with this system in that physicians in this particular emergency department are compensated based on productivity. Taking time to support midlevel providers detracts from personal productivity. So, helping the provider team as a whole comply with hospital policy and provide quality patient care potentially means taking a hit to the "nice" physician's paycheck. Not only does this system discourage physicians and midlevel providers from working cooperatively, barriers to getting the support NPs and PAs may need delays care, results in slower turnover of exam rooms, and ultimately reduces productivity of the overall team.

Regardless of the level of experience of midlevel providers in your practice, effective management is essential for a collegial and efficient work environment. Fostering a positive workplace culture, meeting productivity and quality metrics, and preventing turnover among both physicians and advanced practice providers depends on effective management and recognition of the educational disparities among healthcare providers. Without a structure conducive to midlevel support, the facility as a whole suffers. Effective management of midlevel providers, in contrast, helps NPs and PAs reach the 80–90% benchmark, benefitting individual providers, the healthcare team, and the company as a whole.

WHY EFFECTIVE MANAGEMENT OF MIDLEVEL PROVIDERS IS SO DIFFICULT TO ACHIEVE

Imagine if we approached the mastery of clinical skills in the same way many of our healthcare facilities approach practice management. In such a scenario, the physician would inform the patient that a surgical procedure was required to alleviate a medical condition. Without guidance or training specific to the diagnosis or procedure, the physician would take the patient to the operating room. Physicians are smart, highly capable individuals, so it would be generally accepted by hospital administrators and outsiders that the MD was up to the task.

Once in the OR, the physician would toy with administering the right amount of anesthesia, possibly giving too much and risking the patient's life, or too little, placing the patient in significant pain. Next, the physician would make an incision in what seemed like the correct anatomical location and fumble around inside the body cavity, making a best guess as to the appropriate correction required to fix the patient's problem.

Information about how to carry out the procedure effectively exists; however, since doctors are smart and competent individuals, each individual physician would learn on a trial-and-error basis, patient by patient. Some lessons learned would harm patients. Some would result in success.

While this scenario seems absurd in the clinical setting, medical practice managers and leaders often take this approach. The overwhelming majority of physicians have little or no formal management training, yet are made responsible for leading staff, overseeing practice budgets, and fostering effective workplace cultures. Guidance about carrying out these business practices effectively is available; business schools across the country teach these skills every day, yet we leave it up to our physicians to reinvent the management wheel. Doctors learn leadership and practice management by trial and error with varying degrees of success. Failed attempts are costly.

The medical profession is much more than a clinical skill set. Healthcare is a business. As a whole, physicians are a smart, well-educated, and highly capable group of individuals. Management and leadership skills, however are learned behaviors; they don't come naturally, even to highly capable people. Dr. Keith Gray, founder of the University of Tennessee's Physician Leadership Academy, says "I'll be honest, I learned pretty quickly that there is very little crossover between clinical expertise and administrative effectiveness."[1] Sure, if you are a physician you have likely experienced "wins" in the leadership responsibilities required by your role; however, without training and experience, your team will rarely reach its full potential.

Medical education focuses on patient care with the business and management aspects of operating a medical practice largely ignored. When it comes to working with nurse practitioners and physician assistants, practice management does not capitalize on the potential that midlevel providers have to offer. There are a few ways this manifests itself in the practice setting:

1. Ineffective employee management style and methods;
2. Lack of systems and processes in the clinical setting;
3. Misguided focus or priorities among providers and staff;
4. Poor fiscal mismanagement; and
5. Failure to create innovate solutions in the face of a complex healthcare delivery system.

Let's look at how each of these management mistakes manifests itself in clinical practice, particularly concerning the employment of midlevel providers.

Ineffective Management Styles and Methods

What was your time in medical school and residency like? I suspect that nights with eight or more hours of sleep were nearly nonexistent and that a similar assessment could be made of your social life. Physicians are trained in a somewhat harsh authoritarian system. As medical students and residents, they endure days without sleep and criticism from instructors. Competition and independence are rewarded. Knowingly or not, new physicians often carry this culture with them as they begin their careers. Employees, however, do not respond well to a critical, competitive work environment; it results in high levels of turnover and negative attitudes among staff.

Physicians can fall into other destructive management patterns as well. Fearful of liability concerns, some micromanage midlevel providers, negating the benefits these employees provide the practice. Other physicians do not delegate effectively, keeping too much of the patient care workload and/or practice operations to themselves. Refusal to delegate places stress on the physician and also prevents the practice from reaching its full potential.

Attempts to control midlevel providers by micromanaging or with a competitive or critical work environment are ineffective. They discourage employees from practicing to their fullest scope of practice and individual capabilities. Without business training, physicians often lack the skills to motivate and empower a patient care team. Midlevel providers, in turn, are written off as ineffective or of little value to the practice when management style is really to blame.

One concept that many physicians fail to understand is expressed by Lawrence Appley, former president of the American Management Association: "management is getting things done through others."[2] Too often, physicians remain focused on their own patient care responsibilities rather than taking time out to guide and support the midlevel providers they work with or delegate responsibilities.

Effective Management Styles and Methods

Management and leadership are not defined by a title, level of education, or an attitude. Rather, an effective manager or leader is defined by the things he or she does. In the healthcare setting, this can look like setting aside time for regularly scheduled one-on-one feedback meetings between supervising physicians and midlevel providers or blocking time to demonstrate procedures, to name a few.

As a whole, the healthcare team would accomplish more with active direction from the leading clinician rather than with each individual hyper-focused on his or her own patient panel. Ultimately, productivity of your organization is determined not by what one individual does, but the cumulative effect of the team overall.

Two key components of effective management in your organization are:

1. Maintaining momentum; and
2. Creating a sense of ownership

Maintaining momentum

Accomplishment keeps us motivated in the workplace. Whether charged with heading a committee responsible for a compliance project, or completing a complex patient visit independently, the midlevel providers in your organization must have a sense of achievement based on their work.

Patient care can quickly feel routine. Many providers feel that they are stuck in an endless cycle of visit after visit, day after day. While the job description for a nurse practitioner or physician assistant may change little over their course of employment, much remains that advanced practice providers in your practice can accomplish. As a leader or manager, it's your job to identify areas that need work, attention, or improvement and help the members of your team work toward them.

Set short-term and long-term goals with each individual provider in your practice. These may include clinical skills such as mastery of certain procedures, professional skills such as adopting certain patient communication norms, or administrative tasks and projects. Ensure that you explain the context of the job and why it's important. You aren't simply giving each provider a "to-do" list. Rather, these are items integral to the success of the individual provider and the practice as a whole. In other words, explain the "why" behind the item. Check in with providers either as a group or individually on a weekly basis. What progress has each made toward reaching individual or group goals?

Finally, celebrate accomplishments. Rewarding hard work and a job well done helps maintain the positive momentum you've created for your practice by providing such direction.

Creating a sense of ownership

A sense of ownership is critical to the satisfaction of midlevel providers on your team. In medicine, we tend to refer to ownership in an exclusively financial context. As a manager, however, creating a sense of ownership means something different. Individuals want to belong, to be a part of something bigger than themselves, and to be working toward something as a valued member of a larger group. As a manager, you are in the unique position to facilitate the development of this ownership among NPs and PAs.

Creating a sense of ownership among midlevel providers in your organization begins with a company culture of problem solving. Undoubtedly, midlevel providers in your practice will encounter problems, small and large, on a daily basis. This is an inevitable part of working in healthcare. Encourage providers to be the solution, to take initiative to when it comes to developing solutions. If a patient is upset about the care they received, get the provider's feedback about what can be done. Choose one of the provider's proposed solutions and ask them to execute the plan.

Has a provider come to you with a system or process in your facility that needs improvement? If the issue is something that is indeed a priority, empower the NP or PA to come up with and help implement a solution. The provider then owns the problem and is empowered to solve it. The end result is accomplishment, a sense of belonging and teamwork. Each individual, regardless of title is responsible for the success of the practice.

Lack of Systems and Processes

A nurse practitioner recently shared that on her first day in a new position, the physician who had hired her was off site at administrative meetings. She received an hour or two of EMR orientation from a representative of the vendor, and that was the extent of her onboarding experience. Needless to say, she started her job feeling lost, frustrated, and disconnected—not the recipe for a longstanding employment relationship. A practice protocol for onboarding new providers would have significantly improved her experience and could potentially have prevented quick turnover.

Systems, processes, and protocols are essential for effective management. In the provider world, however, where doctors often chock up their decisions to "clinical judgment," systems, processes, and protocols might as well be four-letter words. Physicians cling to their ability to make decisions independently, but when it comes to management, lack of structure is detrimental to a practice and affects overall productivity.

With systems and processes in place for both clinical and practice operations, healthcare organizations run far more effectively. Fewer errors occur, protecting the practice from liability. Processes also ensure that practices capitalize on reimbursement, allowing individual providers to keep up with the latest billing and coding requirements—an increasingly difficult task given the ever-changing healthcare landscape. Midlevel providers and physicians alike operate more efficiently with a predetermined plan of care or systems in place to guide clinical decision making and daily responsibilities.

Effective Systems and Processes

Implementing systems and processes in your practice can be as simple as creating a checklist. Or, it can include more complex materials like an employment manual or databases of internal company information and metrics. Make sure that all processes are written for easy reference and to ensure compliance and consistency.

When employing midlevel providers, start by having these essential systems in place:

1. Provider credentialing;
2. Employee orientation and onboarding;

3. Midlevel provider training and oversight;
4. Regularly scheduled performance evaluation; and
5. Protocol for handling problems/frustrations.

At initial glance, it may seem that some systems and processes are nearly impossible to implement in some healthcare settings. However, in most cases, practice administrators and clinicians find that with an initial time investment, structure can be created and will result in an overall increase in practice efficiency and therefore revenue.

Misguided Focus/Priorities

As I learned to work as a new nurse practitioner in the emergency department, I was constantly reminded by the department director to "look at the patient, not the monitor." Concerned about a COPD patient with an oxygen saturation far below normal, I would rush over to his work station informing the director of the critical value. "Well, what does the patient look like?" he would ask.

Just as inexperienced clinicians may place inappropriate emphasis on vital signs over patient report and appearance, healthcare management often emphasizes achieving metrics over investing in the individuals who make up the healthcare team. Feedback centers around wait times and CMS scores rather than instruction in the skills necessary to meet these expectations.

Providers must be taught *how* to achieve desired targets, rather than simply given a set of metrics to hit. Providers must also understand the *why* behind what you ask of them. This gives purpose to everyday activities, especially those that may not be particularly popular or enjoyable. Even when providers have the tools, knowledge, and support to achieve such metrics, they are seldom inspired by them. A management style that shields advanced practice providers from practice frustrations like government policies, and instead motivates them to focus on patient care, will improve overall performance and meet expectations. Manage people first, and metrics will follow.

Fiscal Mismanagement

The physician CEO of a clinic client of my company decided he wanted to bring a new nurse practitioner on board his team through Midlevels for the Medically Underserved. He interviewed several applicants to the program and honed in on one NP who seemed to be a particularly good fit for his practice. Bilingual, she could connect with his patient population, not to mention she was Ivy League educated and very personable—the perfect person for the job.

The physician, however, had committed to hiring a midlevel provider before reviewing his budget. So, he dragged his feet when it came to moving forward with this NP's interview and hiring process. As a highly sought-after applicant, this NP accepted another position. Finally, by the time the physician had reviewed his budget, it was too late. He was back at square one, interviewing additional applicants for the job.

This cycle repeated itself several times, with the physician CEO never quite seeming to have a grasp on the financials of his practice. In the end, he missed out on a cost-effective hiring solution through a residency-like program and spent thousands of dollars and hours of his own valuable time on an interview process he wasn't even sure he needed.

The financials associated with operating a medical practice are complex. Third-party payers, for example, make reimbursement for services rendered anything but straightforward. Healthcare facilities operate on large budgets that require experience to manage. Even when budgets are broken down by department, physicians often lack the training to analyze these financials and make educated decisions as to how to allocate funds.

Hiring decisions and assessments about the value advanced practice providers offer are too often made based on a "feeling" rather than hard financial data. Without training in the business and financials of healthcare, physicians may assess staffing structures and decisions incorrectly. Physicians who are considering bringing midlevel providers into the practice should identify an individual with financial know-how to help assess the cost-benefit ratio.

Succumbing to the System

Healthcare delivery is a complex and often defeating system. Without an intimate knowledge of the system and its structure, physicians don't effectively manage midlevel providers or take full advantage of the value they provide.

Rather than blaming the system for workplace woes, practice administrators must develop innovative solutions for working within an inefficient system. They must insulate midlevel providers from the often-demoralizing challenges of working within a bureaucratic healthcare system. For example, providing a transparent, salaried compensation structure can reduce rates of turnover and improve employee satisfaction.

EMPLOYED PHYSICIANS AREN'T OFF THE HOOK

As part of the curriculum for Midlevels for the Medically Underserved, my company's residency-like program for nurse practitioners and physician assistants, I included a presentation on leadership and management as part of the providers' initial training. At the end of the session, several participants commented that the content was interesting but wouldn't apply to them personally. As nurse practitioners, they were focused strictly on patient care and did not have management or administrative ambitions.

A few months later, I began to get calls from individual nurse practitioners in the program. The first call was from Stephanie, a new graduate working in a hospital-based primary care practice. She lamented that her assigned medical assistant constantly entered information incorrectly into patient charts. The assistant arrived late and couldn't keep up with patient flow, meaning that the duo was constantly running behind. She failed to respond to feedback regarding her performance.

The second call was from Elizabeth, a new graduate nurse practitioner working at an outpatient pediatric primary care clinic in California. The two nurses she was assigned to work with had poor attitudes and Elizabeth began dreading work.

I reminded each NP of our leadership presentation, which included tools for handling performance problems. They had mistakenly assumed that as nurse practitioners they had no managerial responsibilities. While they did not employ their medical assistants directly, they did hold a supervisory position and were ultimately responsible for and affected by their performance.

Similarly, physicians who aren't practice owners or who do not hold leadership titles often assume that leadership and management principles are irrelevant in their jobs. In reality, however, these physicians face similar challenges to doctors operating practices independently or with administrative titles. Working with nurse practitioners and physician assistants places physicians in a natural position of leadership within the practice. Advanced practice providers and other practice staff naturally turn to physicians to set the tone of the workplace and to solve problems.

The complex organizational structures of hospitals and large medical practices makes management tricky. Delegating within a hospital hierarchy may not be as straightforward as it seems. In the emergency department where I work, for example, physicians and midlevel providers are employed by an outside group that contracts with the hospital. In the clinical setting, we work alongside nurses, medical assistants, and administrators who are all hospital employees. Physicians may delegate to nurses, however as contracted entities, have little power to make decisions about how the nurse-physician relationship works.

While physicians' ability to see patients is affected by members of hospital staff, when problems with performance arise, they have little recourse, as they are not hospital employees. Effectively managing such employment relationships and navigating contractual constraints requires leadership savvy attained through education and experience.

Many doctors shy away from management and leadership training, preferring a clinically focused career rather than one that involves climbing the healthcare corporate ladder. Clinical practice, however, inherently involves a level of management and leadership. Delegating tasks to other providers and nurses can be done with varying degrees of efficiency and significantly affect a practice's bottom line. Skills for doing so effectively benefit even those physicians who do not have administrative titles. Just like a knowledge of anatomy and physiology is central to the medical profession, so is knowledge of the organizational aspects of healthcare.

HOW PHYSICIANS CAN GET THE MANAGEMENT AND LEADERSHIP EDUCATION THEY NEED

Medical schools increasingly are recognizing the need for the integration of business courses into curriculum, yet the education provided typically is not sufficient.

Recognizing this deficit, some medical students elect to attend one of a growing number of MD/MBA programs to obtain a more well-rounded healthcare education. For most physicians, however, the expense and time required to attend an MBA program is not necessary or justified. Fortunately, there are several options for physicians interested in improving leadership and management skills without such an intense curriculum.

First, physicians may engage in a do-it-yourself style of education. Business books, both those directed to healthcare professionals and those geared toward the corporate world in general, give practical advice for making effective management decisions. I suggest beginning your reading with Ferdinand Fournies' *Coaching for Improved Work Performance*. Medical practice management conferences and conferences for leaders and managers in professional settings also offer helpful advice applicable to the medical practice setting.

More structured options for physicians looking to master medical practice management include a number of non-degree programs for physicians and hospital administrators. The Harvard Business School's Managing Healthcare Delivery Program, for example, consists of three one-week courses spread out over nine months. The program costs $24,000 (2016), and covers topics like Exploring Criteria for High-Performing Hospital Teams and Emphasizing Clinicians as Managers and Leaders. Other universities offer leadership training programs for physicians of varying length and intensity.

OUTSOURCING LEADERSHIP AND MANAGEMENT

Leadership and management skills are essential to day-to-day practice operations. Physicians operating their own practices without a higher level of business education may be best served by outsourcing practice administration responsibilities. Outsourcing administration leaves management and leadership strategy to an individual who specializes in such skills and allows physicians to focus their time and energy on patient care. Operating a medical practice and serving a clinical role can be a difficult balance. Attempting to do both may leave the physician feeling like a failure in each role. Removing the physician, at least partially, from the administrative equation by hiring an outside administrator allows for greater focus on each of the aspects of the practice, ensuring the business succeeds.

The Mayo Clinic is a healthcare institution that has recognized this leadership vacuum in healthcare and has come up with an innovative solution that harnesses the strengths of both physicians and administrators. Physicians at the Mayo Clinic participate in rotating committee assignments where they partner with administrators to develop strategies and give input into organizational decision making. This way, those most involved in the organization's mission—patient care—provide context for the decisions made by the management experts, hospital administrators. The partnership of experienced business leaders with physicians is one of the keys to the Mayo Clinic's success.

IN SUMMARY

Providing training and a support structure to help midlevel providers achieve high levels of productivity requires effective practice management. These skills do not come naturally to physician leaders and must be a conscious pursuit in order to effectively employ midlevel providers to their full potential.

REFERENCES

1. Barnet, S. What they don't teach in medical school: The interesting story behind UTMC's leadership academy. *Becker's Hospital Review.* July 8, 2015. www.beckershospitalreview.com/hospital-management-administration/what-they-don-t-teach-in-medical-school-the-interesting-story-behind-utmc-s-leadership-academy.html. Accessed November 18, 2016.
2. Fournies, F. F. *Coaching for Improved Work Performance.* London: McGraw-Hill; 2000.

CHAPTER 4

Midlevel Providers and Your Practice

Using NPs and PAs to increase revenue and improve work-life balance

The emergency department environment presents several challenges for providers and administrators; it rarely scores highly on patient satisfaction. Prioritizing patients by acuity level leaves stable patients seated in the waiting room for hours, feeling overlooked. Patients leaving the department as a result of long wait times or dissatisfaction with service represents lost revenue.

In the emergency department where I work, administrators closely monitor providers' performance metrics, with time as the primary metric by which performance is evaluated. The length of time a patient sits in the waiting room, the length of time between when the patient is placed in an exam room and when the provider greets the patient, and the amount of time between when the provider sees the patient and when an initial order is placed are all carefully measured and monitored. A focus on such metrics frustrates many providers; catering to the clock seems directly counter to providing quality patient care.

Facing this challenge, one of the emergency departments where I practice found a solution to this frustration in nurse practitioners. A "provider in triage" staffing model places a midlevel provider in the triage room alongside the triage nurse. The provider in triage quickly screens each patient and orders necessary initial testing. This way, patients in the waiting room may have labs drawn and diagnostic imaging performed before an exam room becomes available. These initial actions reassure patients that something is being done to help with their problem, even before the facility can accommodate them in a room. It also ensures that services are rendered in a timely manner and that each patient receives an appropriate medical screening exam.

Since implementing this model, the department's patient satisfaction scores have increased and performance based on time metrics is at an all-time high. Average volumes in the department have steadily increased as a result.

The role the midlevel provider plays in triage in this scenario is not a traditional patient interaction. Rather, it's a quick screening exam. The role also can be somewhat monotonous and was not a role the physicians in the department wanted to play. This solution capitalizes on the value advanced practice providers provide and serves to improve overall department revenue along with patient and provider satisfaction.

Your practice, too, can utilize midlevel providers to increase efficiency and productivity by thinking outside the box.

INCREASE REVENUE WITH MIDLEVEL PROVIDERS

Hiring a midlevel provider over a physician for your practice saves money. According to the U.S. Bureau of Labor Statistics, the mean annual wages for healthcare providers are as follows:[1]

- Family and General Physicians: $192,120
- Nurse Practitioners: $101,260
- Physician Assistants: $99,210

Employing a nurse practitioner or physician assistant, on average, saves a practice between $90,860 and $92,910 in salary alone compared with hiring a physician. In addition, the cost of benefits, employment taxes, and liability coverage costs are also significantly lower for midlevel providers, conferring further savings to a practice.

Recruitment fees, sign-on bonuses, relocation reimbursement, and other financial onboarding expectations are similarly less costly for midlevel providers compared to those of physicians. These fringe benefits can amount to tens of thousands of dollars, realizing even more savings by employing advanced practice providers.

Finally, in many physician practices, MDs are hired as members of the practice group and offered an ownership stake in the practice. Midlevel providers do not expect ownership as part of a compensation package, which is a significant financial benefit to the practice.

Table 4.1 illustrates an estimate of these savings:

TABLE 4.1. Annual Employment Cost Comparison Physician vs. Midlevel Provider

Annual Salary & Benefits	Physician	Midlevel Provider
Salary	$192,120	$101,260
Payroll Taxes, Benefits, PTO*	$38,424	$20,252
Education Allowance	$4,000	$1,500
Malpractice Insurance	$1,700	$900
Bonuses, Profit Sharing, Other Incentives	$ Varies	$0
Total Cost of Employment	$236,244	$123,912
Savings		+$112,332

*Payroll taxes, benefits and PTO/vacation time are estimated at 20% of salary.

The savings associated with NP and PA employment are even more significant in specialty settings or practice settings where physician salaries are higher than those in primary care. Nurse practitioners and physician assistants in specialty settings do command higher salaries than those working primary care, however not to the same extent as physicians.

In a cardiology group, for example, cardiologists may earn salaries of $350,000 to $500,000 or more. NPs and PAs working for the group may expect to earn along the lines of $150,000 or less. This means that extending the manpower of the group with midlevel providers saves the group hundreds of thousands of dollars per NP or PA compared to hiring an additional physician.

MAXIMIZE PERFORMANCE WITH MIDLEVEL PROVIDERS

Working in the fast-track section of the emergency department, there are days when I vow that if I see one more patient with non-emergent chronic back pain, I will lose my mind. Or, I swear that if another patient presents via ambulance for a stubbed toe or broken fingernail, I will toss my computer screen out the proverbial window.

My clinical interests lie in treating patients who are urgently and emergently ill, not with those whose illnesses and injuries barely warrant a visit to a healthcare provider at all, let alone the emergency department. As a midlevel provider, however, part of my role is staffing the low acuity section of the department, freeing up physician time and manpower to treat higher acuity patients.

As healthcare providers, physicians, and advanced practice providers, we all have varied clinical interests and enjoy interacting with different types of patients. As a physician practice owner or leader, hiring a nurse practitioner or physician assistant frees up your time and gives you the flexibility to treat the types of patients that interest you most.

There are a few ways a practice may be structured to maximize time and provider preferences:

1. Assign patients based on acuity or level of complexity;
2. Assign patients based on urgency; and
3. Co-manage patients, assigning each step in the patient care process.

While structuring your practice in such a way that each provider builds his or her own patient panel is a possibility, delegating a specific subset of patients to a midlevel provider can give you as a physician the freedom to focus on a specific clinical area or delegate to maximize the top skills and experience level of each provider.

Structuring Provider Staffing Based on Acuity/Complexity

In practices that structure provider staffing based on level of acuity, physicians treat patients with complex chronic diseases, those with multiple comorbidities, and those of high acuity, while NPs and PAs care for patients with fewer comorbidities and more straightforward clinical presentations. In the primary care setting, for example, a nurse practitioner might treat a patient with relatively well-controlled diabetes and hypertension, while the physician manages a patient with uncontrolled diabetes, hypertension, a history of stroke, and chronic renal failure.

This staffing model works especially well for practices with inexperienced or moderately experienced midlevel providers who may not have the clinical expertise necessary to manage highly complex patients without oversight. Logistically, this model presents some challenges when scheduling patients, as office staff may not be familiar with patients' medical histories or understand which patients qualify as more or less complex. This problem can be solved by implementing a brief question-and-answer protocol for new patients when scheduling appointments.

Delegating patient care responsibilities according to acuity or level of complexity takes advantage of physicians' higher level of clinical knowledge. It allows physicians to spend more time using this specialized clinical skill set, the level of which may or may not have been attained by the nurse practitioner or physician assistant. Many physicians find working with a clinically challenging patient population to be more satisfying, making their jobs more rewarding.

Structuring Provider Staffing Based on Urgency

Some practices capitalize on the value midlevel providers offer by delegating walk-ins, urgent visits, or rounding to NPs and PAs. For example, in the primary care setting, management of patients with chronic disease and most scheduled visits may be delegated to physicians. Patients requiring interim care between appointments or visits for illness or injury may be treated by midlevel providers, as these tend to be more straightforward encounters. For example, a patient might see the physician for management and follow up of diabetes, hypertension, and Parkinson's Disease. When the patient experiences a fall related to his Parkinson's, the midlevel provider treats the patient for the injury.

This staffing structure permits physicians to maintain full schedules while still allowing the practice to accommodate patients with unscheduled problems. This model keeps patients turning to the practice when needs arise rather than relying on the increasing number of urgent care or retail health clinics or heading to the emergency department. It also prevents providers from feeling overwhelmed and overworked. Patients with urgent needs are directed to a controlled system to receive care rather than worked into a provider's already-packed schedule. The latter method makes wait times longer for patients and is a recipe for provider burnout.

Finally, for physicians who prefer to manage chronic disease or complex patients rather than those with acute illnesses, injuries or less complex problems, this model delegates patient care responsibilities accordingly.

Staffing with a Co-management Model

In some settings, patients are co-managed by both a physician and advanced practice providers. Pieces of the patient care process are delegated specifically to each type of provider. Most commonly, this model is integrated into specialty practices and the inpatient hospital setting, although it can be effective in other areas as well.

One of my former nurse practitioner school classmates works within this staffing structure in rural Tennessee, where there are few healthcare resources for patients in her area, especially when it comes to specialty care. So, a larger oncology group in a nearby urban area has placed a small clinic in this outlying town. An oncologist visits the town just once a week, seeing new patients and prescribing appropriate chemotherapy regimens. The remainder of the week, a solo NP oversees chemo administration and treats patients for complications and side effects of treatment as well as other problems that arise. The model is cost effective and capitalizes on the skill sets of each type of provider.

Ultimately, implementing a staffing model with midlevel providers allows practices to add manpower in a cost-effective manner. It frees up time for physicians to interact with the subset of patients they enjoy most. By capitalizing on the strengths of physicians, as well as the benefits that come with employing midlevel providers, job satisfaction increases, leading to an improved patient experience.

MIDLEVEL PROVIDERS MAKE LOWER-RISK HIRES

There's a lot at stake when hiring a physician to join a practice. Many groups require a "buy-in" for the new physician and confer an ownership stake in the practice as part of an employment package. Even if the physician does not acquire a piece of the group, profit sharing and other complex compensation models are likely involved in hiring an MD. The new member may gain a vote in matters that pertain to the structure and organization of the practice. This affects practice financials, group dynamics, and how the business operates.

With so much on the line, smart physician groups spend a significant amount of time, energy, and finances on the hiring process. A physician who doesn't contribute positively to the group, underperforms, or is a divisive member of the team, is difficult to get rid of once he or she is tied to the practice with an ownership stake.

In contrast to hiring a physician, bringing on an advanced practice provider is a low-risk and relatively simple process. Nurse practitioners and physician assistants don't expect to have ownership in a practice or profit-sharing benefits. As a result, in most groups, they will not have an equivalent vote in decisions affecting organizational structure. While this may or may not be the most effective way to operate a practice, in reality, most practices are hierarchical with physicians in administrative seats.

Given these realities, nurse practitioners and physician assistants represent a straightforward way for your practice to increase patient volume and fill provider vacancies without the complexities associated with bringing on a physician. If the NP or PA is not a culture fit for your practice or does not meet expectations, cutting ties is a much simpler process.

MIDLEVEL PROVIDERS PROVIDE
ORGANIZATIONAL STABILITY

I spoke recently with Brian, the CEO of a rural hospital in New Mexico. Plagued with staffing problems given the hospital's location, Brian lamented that he was at the mercy of the facility's physicians. A single physician leaving a hospital department or affiliated outlying clinic left a gaping hole in the facility's ability to see patients. He was held hostage by those demanding higher salaries in order to stay. A rural health budget didn't allow Brian to solve his problem by creating multi-physician departments or even by awarding financial incentives to doctors. Instead, he came up with an innovative but simple solution.

Brian hired a nurse practitioner to work alongside and support each specialty physician. These NPs were trained to practice to the highest level possible under the physician in that specialty. An extra set of hands increased patient volume and thereby revenues.

Additionally, when a physician left the facility, a capable provider was available to fill in the gap and maintain the department in the absence of the physician. Yes, in some settings such as surgical specialties, the NP could not fill the shoes of the physician completely; however, follow-up appointments and referrals could fill the gap during the search for a new doctor. No longer was the department brought to a grinding halt.

Providers leave practices. Patient volumes wax and wane with season, time, or for seemingly no reason at all. Preparing for such organizational variables by employing additional physicians is costly. Using NPs and PAs as a buffer to accommodate busy seasons or to fill employment gaps is a financially feasible solution. Planning ahead by employing midlevel providers gives your organization stability, helping you stay afloat when things don't go as planned.

IMPROVE WORK-LIFE BALANCE
WITH MIDLEVEL PROVIDERS

Sitting at my station in the ED, I often observe hospitalists with wonder. "Why would anyone sign up for that job?" I think silently to myself, "It just may be the worst job in the world." Working seven-in-a-row strings of 12-hour shifts, often overnight, the physical demands of the position alone are high, not to mention the fact that constant admissions means managing many patients simultaneously. It's no wonder MDs lament their skewed work-life balance.

As a physician, you know what it's like to feel off-balance when it comes to your career and personal life. On-call commitments force you to decline social engagements. Your pager vibrates, beeps, and buzzes at all hours of the night. Your specialty may require working on weekends and/or holidays. The intrusion, and even simply the threat of the intrusion of work into your daily life outside of the clinic or hospital walls is stressful. It affects your friendships, your family, your physical health, and your mood. Remedying the problem means taking time out for yourself, but your erratic schedule doesn't allow for time away. The responsibilities and demands of your position weigh heavily on you. You are a slave to your job.

Fortunately, there is solution: delegate. While midlevel providers aren't interested in signing up for misaligned work-life balance either, sharing responsibilities translates to more freedom for each provider in the group. Depending on state scope of practice laws and the skill level of the NPs and PAs you work with, backup call may still be required. However, at the very least, an advanced practice provider can field initial calls and filter them so only those that truly require your attention reach your cell phone.

A similar principle applies for physicians burned out from working holidays, weekends, and too many hours in general. Employing midlevel providers spreads out staffing in a cost-effective manner. Some clinics even delegate weekend shifts solely to NPs and PAs. Sharing this responsibility among a greater number of providers allows you more time for family and leisure, tipping the work-life balance scale to a more neutral position.

PREVENT BURNOUT WITH NPS AND PAS

Burnout is a buzzword these days in the healthcare community and may be met with an eye roll by some, but the phenomenon is a reality for doctors. Working as a healthcare provider is stressful and demanding. Your group or employer places demands on you, patients place demands on you, all the while the government and insurance companies place demands on you, making it impossible to please everyone. The loss of control over the way you practice, coupled with an excessive workload, is a recipe for feeling overwhelmed.

More physicians than ever are feeling the effects of burnout. A 2015 Mayo Clinic study showed that over 50% of U.S. physicians experience at least one symptom of burnout, an increase of 20% over 2011 survey results.[2] Medscape's 2013 Physician Lifestyle Report surveyed physicians who identified the top causes of burnout as:[3]

1. Too many bureaucratic tasks;
2. Spending too many hours at work;
3. Present and future impact of the Patient Protection and Affordable Care Act;
4. Feeling like "just a cog in the wheel"; and
5. Income not high enough.

The good news? Remedying the majority of these burnout-causing issues is within the physician's control. Along similar lines to improving work-life balance, one solution for curbing burnout is employing NPs and PAs.

Bureaucratic tasks suck the joy out of patient care and the passion out of practicing medicine. Spending excess hours on the job has a similar effect. Dealing with these aspects of healthcare quickly leads to frustration and ultimately burnout. While you can't influence the hoops that payers make you jump through or the bureaucratic demands of a large hospital system, you can control the way you approach them. Bringing more hands on deck allows you to delegate some of these tasks and workload, freeing you from the burnout burden.

In most states, the scope of practice for nurse practitioners and physician assistants is such that these providers can take on the majority of the paperwork and patient care responsibilities required of physicians. So, offload a share of these duties by hiring a midlevel provider to ease your workload. This restores your ability to spend adequate time with patients bringing meaning back to your work.

Related to income, not only can working with NPs and PAs improve practice revenues, it allows physicians to focus on activities that generate higher rates of reimbursement, capitalizing on the strengths of both midlevel providers and their own skills as a physician. With a midlevel provider on board to follow up with patients in the clinic or round on patients in the hospital, a specialist, for example, may free up time to perform more advanced procedures or surgeries. Performing more procedures generates more revenue leading to a better income or an equivalent income earned in fewer hours.

I'VE TRIED IT AND IT DOESN'T WORK...

You may be thinking, "I've tried, and it doesn't work." I often talk with physicians, CMOs, and CEOs who are in your shoes who have hired a "lemon" of a midlevel provider in the past who wasn't a fit for the practice culture, causing the company to stray from this model of care. Or, maybe physicians in the practice have a stigma against midlevel providers and haven't accepted their implementation into the practice. Perhaps you have hired a less-experienced NP or PA and weren't prepared for the amount of clinical support that would be required in the initial months of employment.

It's true, nurse practitioners and physician assistants are not the solution to every practice woe. And, if mismanaged, they are not the solution to any practice woe. In the same way that you regularly service technical equipment used in your practice, you must maintain the human assets of your practice: your employees. Maximizing the value nurse practitioners and physician assistants provide depends on the manner in which they are managed. You must put time, thought, and energy into the employment relationship for it to succeed.

If you employ midlevel providers and you are not enjoying the benefits described in this chapter, the techniques outlined in the following chapters will help turn your practice around.

REFERENCES

1. U.S. Department of Labor Bureau of Labor Statistics. Occupational Employment and Wages, May 2015; Family and General Practitioners. Bureau of Labor Statistics Web site. www.bls.gov/oes/current/oes291062.htm. Accessed November 4, 2016.
2. Shanafelt TD, MD, Hasan O., MBBS, MPH, & Dyrbye LN, MD. Changes in burnout and satisfaction with work-life balance in physicians and the general US working population between 2011 and 2014. *Mayo Clin Proc.,2015;* 90(12):1600-1613.
3. Peckham C. Physician lifestyles—Linking to burnout: A Medscape survey. Medscape Web site. www.medscape.com/features/slideshow/lifestyle/2013/public#1. Accessed October 4, 2016.

CHAPTER 5

Nurse Practitioners and Training

What happens when things go right

I n some cases, you may hire a midlevel provider and hit the jackpot. The provider fits in with the culture of your practice, works efficiently, has significant clinical experience and a skill set to show for it. In other cases, you may find that a provider, experienced or otherwise, fails to meet expectations. This leads to frustration and dissatisfaction with the employment arrangement.

Nurse practitioners and physician assistants receive the majority of their training on the job. If prior experience does not match up directly with responsibilities of the current position, without proper training, the provider will most certainly fail to meet expectations. How can you as an employer or supervising physician set nurse practitioners and physician assistants up for success?

CORRECTING MISGUIDED ASSUMPTIONS

Physicians complete years of intense training after medical school in a residency and possibly a fellowship. Family medicine physicians, for example, undergo three rigorous years of residency after graduating from a four-year medical school program. Nurse practitioners and physician assistants, on the other hand, receive significantly less training as part of their education, usually in a two-year master's level program.

Nurse practitioners receive on average around 700 hours of experience in the clinical setting as part of an NP program. This equates to about 18 weeks of full-time work experience. It is generally accepted that midlevel providers working in the primary care setting, however, can perform about 80% of the job responsibilities of a physician. The knowledge and skills conferred by a physician's three-year or longer residency, however, cannot possibly be attained by a nurse practitioner with fewer than five months of full-time clinical training. Given these educational disparities, it seems obvious that on-the-job training would be a necessity for NPs and PAs.

I recently talked with Lynn, the human resources director of a primary care system in San Diego, about her facility's staffing situation. She recounted her experiences with new graduate NPs and PAs, both positive and negative. Lynn recalled the facility's mistake with one inexperienced NP. The provider was an excellent culture fit for the practice, passionate about primary care and the population the clinic served. The clinic sensed her eagerness and delegated to her some administrative tasks in addition to her clinical work.

"It did not go well," Lynn said. The inexperienced NP was unable to balance time spent honing her skills as a clinician with the administrative tasks she had been delegated. "We misjudged her abilities and put too much on her too early." Lynn regretted the decision, as it resulted in what could have been a long-term employment relationship ending on a sour note.

Employers often make the mistake of hiring midlevel providers, particularly newer graduates, with the assumption that they are fully prepared for their role. The provider is immediately expected to take on a full panel of patients and treat individuals with complex medical conditions or with high acuity problems. Ill-equipped to handle such patients, the midlevel provider requires frequent assistance. If a framework is not in place for providing this support, other providers' work schedules are disrupted by the additional responsibility of assisting the new midlevel provider.

Facilities that don't have adequate staff to provide support and mentoring place patients in unsafe situations and leave the midlevel provider unable to render necessary care. This not only exposes the facility legally, but also sets the stage for job dissatisfaction and turnover among NPs, PAs, and other staff members.

Neglecting to provide adequate training and support to nurse practitioners and physician assistants burdens the practice as a whole. Staffing and practice culture suffer without proper onboarding and follow-up, and lead to turnover, which has a trickle-down effect as existing work is redistributed, placing an additional burden on remaining providers. If instability in the practice persists for too long, providers become dissatisfied.

Nurses, medical assistants, and staff may also grow frustrated with the unstable practice structure. The time required to recruit, interview, and hire additional providers and staff detracts from other managerial and patient care responsibilities. Patient care and productivity suffer as a result of turnover and burnout, ultimately impacting practice revenues.

The assumption that a practice can hire a midlevel provider and provide little training and support is most often misguided and sets the employment relationship up for failure. Nurse practitioners and physician assistants gain a foundational understanding of medicine in their educational programs; however, the time NPs and PAs spend on their education is insufficient for initial success in the "real-life" clinical environment.

If expectations of the employer are not set accordingly, the employment arrangement can send the practice into a downward spiral. A plan to onboard, train, mentor, and support midlevel providers is essential to attaining the benefits that NPs and PAs offer.

RECOGNIZING THE TENSION OF
PATIENT CARE + TRAINING

Recently, I spoke with a family nurse practitioner named Brenda. Brenda has a background in nursing, including seven years of experience in the ICU, but is a recent NP graduate and new to the provider role. She had worked for her most recent employer for three months.

Dr. Riggens, the physician who hired her, owns a busy primary care practice and maintains his own patient panel. With a packed schedule, Dr. Riggens quickly became overwhelmed by training Brenda. Rather than taking time out of his schedule to assist her or allow her to job shadow as an onboarding strategy, he relegated Brenda to documenting and entering patient orders into the computer to expedite patient care. Brenda functioned as a scribe and glorified secretary rather than a clinician.

While Dr. Riggens' frustration was understandable, his answer to the problem proved to be the proverbial shot in the foot. His solution did not maximize Brenda's potential. An initial time investment in her training would have meant another billing provider on the practice's team. It would also have alleviated some of Dr. Riggens' own overwhelming patient load. Instead, he essentially created a position for an overpaid assistant.

Frustrated that she was not functioning in her role as a provider, Brenda left the practice. The lack of training and support offered at the clinic landed Dr. Riggens squarely back in the demanding process of recruiting, hiring, and onboarding another provider—a job arguably as time consuming as training Brenda would have been in the first place.

One of the most common reasons nurse practitioners leave their jobs is lack of clinical support. Management and training of advanced practice providers is time intensive and often can only be accomplished by another billing provider. Physicians sacrificing time from their own schedules to train and manage midlevel providers, for example, may notice a temporary drop in their own productivity. Too often, medical practices make the mistake of prioritizing short-term revenue over the more profitable decision to take the time to train nurse practitioners and physician assistants effectively.

Employers, especially those who are also physicians, must maintain a longer-term perspective when it comes to decisions about hiring and onboarding. Taking time out of one's own billable patient encounters to train and support midlevel providers means lost revenue. Investing this time into another provider, however, quickly becomes worth the effort. As the competency of the NP or PA increases, productivity naturally follows. The time commitment required to support the nurse practitioner or physician assistant gradually decreases. The initial financial setback is quickly outweighed by having another provider on board to share in patient care responsibilities.

Finally, adequate training and support stops the cycle of provider turnover. Turnover is costlier than training. Turnover requires that, once again, the physician or administrative team member takes time from his or her own schedule to train the replacement. It is to a practice's financial advantage to retain a provider who may require training rather than risk turnover. Turnover equates to a vacancy, potentially for months, resulting in tens of thousands of dollars or more in missed revenue.

While training and managing nurse practitioners and physician assistants is time intensive, physicians must realize that they are indirectly compensated for midlevel providers' work. The big picture must be taken into account. Investing in the success of the NPs and PAs on your team means investing in the success of the practice as a whole.

WHAT DOES SUPPORTING A MIDLEVEL PROVIDER LOOK LIKE?

Training, mentoring, and supporting a midlevel provider in the clinical setting includes four main components:

1. Responding to questions;
2. Observation;
3. Clinical training; and
4. Patient panel selection.

When I was a nurse practitioner new to the emergency department, one physician recognized the importance of these components. To this day, I attribute my success and longevity as an ED provider to his efforts to train me.

Responding to questions

When the department was slow, or I didn't have quite enough patients to keep me busy, the physician would stroll over to my desk and say, "Come on! Let's go see patients." I followed him around the department observing how he interacted with patients and made clinical decisions. He taught me and quizzed me, never in a condescending manner. As questions arose throughout my shift, he paused to not only answer them, but also to walk with me into the patient's room to make sure I was on the right track.

Typically, midlevel providers require support from physicians and other more experienced providers in the form of availability to answer questions during daily patient encounters. The time commitment of this responsibility depends on the extent of the midlevel provider's experience in the particular clinical setting. Inexperienced providers, for example, may initially have questions about the majority of patients they treat. More experienced midlevel providers may rarely require assistance, relying primarily on outside resources when questions arise.

Observation

Direct observation is an important and often neglected component of clinical training. Inexperienced NPs and PAs will benefit significantly by observing the way other providers practice. This exposes the provider to more complex patients who can be used as learning opportunities. It helps providers new to the practice become familiar with day-to-day facility operations. Observation may occur during downtime in the midlevel provider's schedule or as a regularly structured learning opportunity.

Clinical training

Given the limited number of clinical hours included in their education programs, inexperienced NPs and PAs benefit from additional clinical training, particularly when it comes to performing hands-on procedures. Expose these providers to as many hands-on opportunities as possible. This helps the NP or PA grow in competence and confidence, leading to autonomy.

Patient panel selection

Finally, assigning patients intentionally helps advanced practice providers succeed and grow. Less-experienced midlevel providers may be assigned a lighter patient load, allowing time for questions and the use of resources to guide patient care without falling behind schedule.

For example, many facilities start new graduates with seeing one patient per hour. Salaries for these inexperienced providers are lower than for those taking on a full patient load, so this structure doesn't have the financial impact on the practice one might anticipate.

Delegating the care of lower acuity patients to new midlevel providers also helps providers gradually improve their clinical skills. Adjust the volume and acuity of patients assigned to midlevel providers to be more challenging as they become more autonomous.

This sounds like a lot of work, but your investment is worth the time and effort. Later, we'll also discuss a compensation model that accounts for the level of experience, clinical skills, and scope of responsibility among midlevel providers in your practice.

The physician who took an interest in overseeing my professional growth in the emergency department was eventually promoted to become the medical director. After making several positive improvements in the department, he was recruited by another facility to turn their department around as well. Wanting to infuse new energy into the ED, he asked if I would join him. Recalling all that he had done for me and looking back on our good working relationship, I accepted and was able to repay the favor—with minimal training necessary in my new position. What goes around comes around.

MUTUALLY BENEFICIAL SUPPORT STRUCTURE

Each of the emergency departments in which I have worked takes a different approach to delegating midlevel supervision responsibilities. One operates with a blanket policy that physicians are to assist NPs and PAs as needed. Midlevel providers direct questions to the physician of their choosing throughout the course of each shift. Consequently, physicians perceived as more approachable end up with greater responsibility.

Another emergency department takes a more effective approach. Each physician is responsible for supervising midlevel providers for a specified number of hours each shift. For the first few hours of the work day, NPs and PAs direct questions to an assigned physician. The latter half of the work day, they direct questions to a different physician. This way, the time commitment associated with supporting midlevel providers does not fall on a single physician and is split equally among MDs.

An effective support system must not only take relationships with midlevel providers into account, but also consider the physicians involved. A vascular surgeon friend of mine, Chris, works for a large group that staffs multiple area hospitals. Relationships among MDs in the group have been tense at times. For Chris, one such frustration arose in the way nurse practitioners are employed in the group.

Each NP is assigned to assist two physicians. These physicians delegate to the NP, who helps manage heavy patient loads, essential for maintaining some semblance of work-life balance among the surgeons. Chris' colleague dominates their shared nurse practitioner's time. Chris is not able to get the support intended from the NP, so the additional workload falls on him. Meanwhile, his colleague enjoys a greater portion of the benefits the NP provides. A system for delegating work is not clearly laid out in the group, allowing for imbalances and the resulting job dissatisfaction.

Intentionally structuring the way training and coaching are offered to midlevel providers in your practice as well as how work is delegated mitigates frustration and minimizes the time commitment. A number of techniques help with successful training and support of midlevel medical providers in your practice.

Schedule coaching sessions

Supporting a midlevel provider can be an unpredictable task. Being approached to answer questions or provide assistance throughout the work day can be disruptive to the supporting provider's schedule and to patient flow. Some clinics have daily or weekly mentoring sessions with new midlevel providers. In these sessions, the midlevel provider anticipates the clinical questions he or she might have and is able to address non-urgent issues. This way, much of the coaching relationship takes place on a predictable schedule.

One of the facilities participating in my company's residency-like program for nurse practitioners and physician assistants excels in this area. Catherine, the new graduate NP paired with the facility, is motivated and smart, but inexperienced. So, the physician medical director of the facility, Dr. Kevin, blocks his schedule from 10:30 a.m. to 11:00 a.m. every day to meet with Catherine. During this time, she anticipates questions she will have about care for her patients. She reviews with him any lab result she isn't sure about. She asks questions about previous visits that were not urgent enough to require immediate attention. This system allows both of their days to flow in a more predictable manner and helps overall practice efficiency.

Keep in mind that with each of these methods, availability of a more experienced provider for issues that arise throughout the clinical day may still be a necessary resource for the inexperienced midlevel provider.

Delegate coaching responsibilities

Spreading the responsibility of supporting a midlevel provider among multiple experienced clinicians prevents a single provider from becoming overwhelmed or burned out. This approach also gives the midlevel provider the experience of working with multiple clinicians practicing from different perspectives.

If you plan to delegate midlevel supervision responsibilities, create a clear plan for doing so to prevent resentment on the part of physicians assigned the responsibility. Outline who will take responsibility for supporting midlevel providers in your practice, when this will happen, and what it entails. Setting clear expectations for providing support and training ensures that the arrangement is fair and that training and support occur in an effective manner.

PITFALLS IN TRAINING

Having worked for nearly three years as a nurse practitioner in the emergency department, Emily was comfortable in her role and had gained the respect and confidence of her physician coworkers. One evening, she encountered a patient whose diagnosis she was not entirely comfortable making. Lab tests and imaging studies all returned falling within normal limits. However, the patient's history of present illness along with his long list of chronic medical problems gave her pause. Concerned she was missing something, she asked her assigned supervising physician to pay the patient a visit as well.

Emily's supervising physician that day did not particularly enjoy supporting the midlevel providers on staff. He preferred to work independently and made his preference known with a subtle eye roll or a tone of annoyance in his voice when asked a question. In this instance, he asked Emily a few questions about the patient rather than making the effort to see the patient himself as she requested.

Based on Emily's responses, the physician determined that it seemed reasonable to send the patient home from the emergency department. She made a note of her discussion with the physician in the patient's chart and allowed the patient to go home. He returned to the emergency department later that evening with a potentially serious complication that might have been detected sooner, had the physician taken the time and made the effort to be a better support system.

Fortunately, in this case, the patient did not have a negative outcome. However, the scenario was a wake-up call to the physician that managing midlevel providers must be taken seriously. The stakes of the responsibility are too high to take the task lightly.

Working with and managing midlevel medical providers, especially those with little experience, isn't for everyone. Time, effort, and an adjustment of one's own patient care responsibilities is required. Managing midlevel providers with a negative attitude or misguided methods is counterproductive to the benefits of hiring these providers.

If physicians are *not* interested in this type of training or mentoring, then hiring an NP or PA is probably not the best decision for your practice, as it won't guarantee maximal benefit. Or, your practice may need to consider only very experienced candidates for its roles.

DESIGNATING THE BEST GO-TO
FOR MIDLEVEL PROVIDERS

An administrative title or an MD behind your name does not necessarily make you the best go-to for NPs and PAs in your practice. Administrative duties coupled with patient care responsibilities may mean you lack the time required to train and coach a midlevel provider. Lack of passion for mentoring and teaching may also mean the task is best delegated to another experienced provider in your practice. Or, your practice may be best served by hiring only experienced NPs and PAs, or without hiring midlevel providers at all.

Entering into the employment relationship dragging your feet is counterproductive for both parties, ensuring the practice will not reap the maximum benefits that midlevel providers have to offer.

While you may not be the appropriate go-to for midlevel providers in your practice, this doesn't preclude you from hiring NPs and PAs altogether. Another physician, experienced NP or PA, or both, may be up for the task.

Training and coaching nurse practitioners and physician assistants, particularly those with less experience, can be quite rewarding. Mentorship comes with a sense of giving back and provides richness and purpose to one's career. Training an NP or PA also requires continued learning on the part of the experienced provider. Defending one's actions in the clinical setting requires a knowledge of the latest treatment and diagnostic guidelines.

If you would like to take advantage of the benefits a midlevel provider can provide but aren't the person for the job, present the opportunity to other qualified providers. Consider making willingness to mentor other providers a component of the compensation levels document outlined in Chapter 6, financially rewarding those who are up for the responsibility.

BEST PRACTICES FOR MANAGING MIDLEVEL PROVIDERS

Practices make several common mistakes in their efforts to onboard and employ nurse practitioners and physician assistants. Finding ways to mitigate these challenges as well as ways to motivate midlevel providers sets the stage for a productive employment relationship.

Correcting behavior

Working triage in the emergency department can be challenging. Patients aren't feeling well and are naturally anxious about wait times. Triage nurses are in the unpopular position of serving as gatekeepers to ensure that the most critical patients are first in line for treatment.

To vent frustration, or in an effort to add some lightheartedness to the work day, some nurses in my department routinely placed comments about patients in the "notes" section of the emergency department patient tracker. These comments were sarcastic and certainly unprofessional.

I'm not against having a little fun on the job, but typing negative comments into a patient's chart, even if not as part of the permanent record, is certainly not professional, even if they are ultimately deleted. You never know who is watching and what may or may not accidentally become part of a patient's permanent record. Should a clinical error or malpractice allegation be made regarding the patient's care, the nurse's comments would undoubtedly be made public and potentially have a disastrous effect on the outcome of the resolution.

What's more, as a provider, I don't like my impression of a patient to be negatively colored before I walk in the room. My initial impression was that these nurses had poor attitudes about their jobs and were negligent about their work performance.

As a nurse practitioner inherently in somewhat of a managerial role over nurses, I was concerned about the situation. So, I expressed my thoughts to the triage nurses directly. The nurses hadn't considered the issue from the provider's perspective and immediately realized their actions may have serious legal implications. They respected how their choices affected me professionally as well. The comments stopped and the (mostly) lighthearted atmosphere we maintain at work was not sacrificed.

Coaching employees to modify their behaviors to benefit the business is at the core of management. Physicians managing midlevel providers must intentionally coach NPs and PAs to work in a way that benefits the practice.

Frustration often arises when the midlevel provider approaches problems or patient care differently than the supervising physician. When a managing physician becomes frustrated, the natural tendency is to blame the midlevel provider, blame midlevel providers as a group, or discount the abilities of the NP or PA. Dissatisfaction with the midlevel provider mounts until the employer-employee relationship has gone sour, propagating the cycle of turnover.

Fortunately, pinpointing the root cause of the problem is often enough to stop this cycle, resolve differences, and help the midlevel provider meet the expectations of the supervising physician.

Physicians and administrators must operate under the assumption that employees want to excel. These employees may behave inappropriately or inefficiently because they don't realize their behavior is an issue or they lack clarity about how to solve the problem. As managers and leaders, we cannot assume the employees who don't measure up are lazy, sloppy, or have poor attitudes.

The trick to leading more effectively? Let the employee know his or her behavior is a problem. Behaviors or issues that seem obvious to you may not be obvious to your employees. Feedback and open communication are essential to the success of nurse practitioners and physician assistants in your practice.

Facilitating behavior change

In addressing performance issues or when training NPs and PAs in general, a key component is often missed in the interaction: Employers must not only inform midlevel providers when performance fails to meet expectations, but also offer the information and tools necessary to change the behavior. Letting the provider know the *what* and *why* of a problem must be accompanied by a *how*.

A nurse practitioner recently contacted me out of frustration. After three months of employment with the clinic where she worked, she was advised that she needed to improve her performance. She was not as productive as other providers, meaning she fell at the bottom of the list when it came to the number of patients she treated and her visits were the lengthiest of the provider group.

Motivated to improve, she worked harder. She asked for feedback from her physician employer several times and was told she was "OK." Then, one day, she was called into her employer's office and notified the practice was terminating her employment.

Despite this nurse practitioner's perceived efforts toward improvement, the metrics by which her employer measured her performance showed no demonstrable improvement. She was frustrated because her managing physician had not offered advice as to *how* to meet these metrics.

Concrete, actionable advice related to documenting efficiently and completing a patient history and physical exam more quickly would have improved this NP's visit times and overall productivity. Instead, the feedback she received was simply that she needed to work more quickly and be more productive. Simply performing her current, flawed practice methods to a greater degree did not equate to the necessary changes. It did not address the root of the problem: a lack of strategies to achieve efficiency. So, what could have been a positive, stable employment relationship with a coachable, motivated midlevel provider ended.

In essence, it was though the employer were telling someone who bikes as a hobby, like me, to beat Lance Armstrong by "going faster." It simply wouldn't work. Without proper equipment, technical instruction, and coaching, I would be nowhere.

As a manager, making employees guess what you are looking for is ineffective. They will miss the mark. Set clear expectations. When providers fail to meet these metrics, offer tangible steps to improve performance. Generalized feedback about working harder, working faster, seeing more patients, or reducing wait times is unlikely to be effective. Identifying the problem alone rather than addressing the root causes of the problem will not lead to the desired changes.

Reinforcing growth and achievement

The urgent care clinic where I worked in my second year of practice housed an ancient X-ray machine. With just the right touch, it remained operational, producing skeletal images on films. Operating on a limited budget, the clinic had no intention of transitioning to a more modern machine with digital X-ray images. An older gentleman regularly visited the clinic to tweak the machine and check radiation levels to keep the ancient piece of equipment operational.

In the same way that medical practices attend to expensive equipment and resources, employees require routine maintenance and attention. As a supporting physician or administrator, you are responsible for the satisfaction and training of midlevel medical providers. Very few medical practices prioritize the opportunity for regular feedback, the basis for providing such support.

Many healthcare providers, midlevel providers included, sense their careers growing stagnant once a certain level of clinical proficiency is accomplished. Unlike the business world, there are few opportunities for providers in patient-facing roles to "move up." In medicine, however, there is always more to learn, and with encouragement even midlevel providers who are clinically advanced have the opportunity to add increasing value to a practice. Training and supporting nurse practitioners and physician assistants doesn't end when a baseline level of competency and confidence is reached.

Depending on the number of your direct reports, set up a schedule by which you give and receive feedback from the NPs and PAs on your team. When an issue arises, you may need to give feedback much more frequently until a resolution is reached. Reinforce achievements such as meeting desired metrics or improving clinical skills. Maintaining an open conversation and forum for communication keeps frustrations from mounting for both parties and serves as a motivational tool.

If you're struggling for a starting point in your feedback conversations, begin by structuring meetings around four questions:

1. Is there anything I/we could be doing more of?
2. Is there anything I/we could be doing less of?
3. Is there anything I/we are doing that you wish I/we were not doing?
4. Is there anything I/we are not doing that you wish we were doing?

The advanced practice provider can give feedback related to his or her work experience and you as a manager can give feedback related to the advanced practice provider's performance within the context of these questions.

TAILORING TRAINING AND SUPPORT TO THE INDIVIDUAL

Employing advanced practice providers and providing training and support are not mutually exclusive. Regardless of the NP's or PA's level of experience, some level of support is required. Even midlevel providers working autonomously face challenges or have room for improvement and growth by learning from other experienced providers. In most states, some form of collaboration or supervisory relationship between an NP or PA and physician is required by law.

The amount of training and support required varies based on the provider's level of experience and the type of setting in which the NP or PA practices. Midlevel providers working in high acuity settings, for example, may require more mentorship. NPs and PAs transitioning to new practice areas may require additional training if prior clinical experience does not translate directly to the new setting.

Invest in the members of your team, even if they seem to get the job done. Regular feedback sessions and education maintain qualify and ensure job satisfaction.

Inexperienced Midlevel Providers

Recent nurse practitioner and physician assistant graduates have a baseline clinical knowledge and very limited experience with hands-on patient care in the provider role. The NP/PA education is not sufficient to prepare these individuals to be comfortable and confident with a number of the clinical scenarios they will encounter daily in most settings.

Facilities that hire recent graduates may consider creating an environment conducive to the success of the new midlevel provider by setting the following expectations:

- Reasonable metrics—Less-experienced providers must interrupt patient care to seek assistance or use resources to help guide clinical decision making. These activities require time. As a result, less-experienced providers should be assigned a lower patient volume that grows as the provider's competency increases.
- Access to experience—Inexperienced midlevel providers must have access to the knowledge and insight of more experienced providers. Ideally, the new NP or PA will work on site with one or more seasoned providers willing to assist as needed, rather than as the sole provider in a department or facility.
- Assign patients intentionally—Assigning lower acuity, more straightforward patients to the inexperienced NPs and PAs facilitates development of baseline competencies in the initial months of practice. As clinical knowledge grows, gradually assign patients with a more complex clinical picture to the new provider.
- Procedural assistance—Nurse practitioner programs notoriously lack procedural training as well as education in interpreting diagnostic tests such as ECGs and X-rays. Expect that experienced providers working alongside the NP will need to teach these skill sets.

While employing inexperienced NPs and PAs requires significant onboarding and support, the relationship does confer several advantages to the employer. These may include:

- Adaptability—Inexperienced midlevel providers don't need to unlearn bad habits. They are more amenable to working in a manner that fits well with the practice environment and structure you have worked hard to create.
- Motivation—New graduate nurse practitioners are eager to perform. They want to do well in their first position, setting a solid foundation for the rest of their career. A positive attitude can overcome the inconvenience of supporting a new graduate through the transition from education to clinical practice. New graduates may be willing to take on tasks other providers may not want or to pick up less-desirable shifts to gain experience. While healthcare providers who have been in practice for many years often become burned out, those with less experience expend more energy toward their careers.
- Changing face of healthcare—Our healthcare delivery system itself is undergoing an overhaul. Providers who are stuck in their ways may fight these changes rather than

adapt to them to the detriment of your practice. New graduates are more amenable to adapting to new healthcare rules, regulations, and legislation as well as developing a practice style that accommodates change on a larger scale.

Experienced Midlevel Providers

Hiring experienced nurse practitioners and physician assistants has the obvious advantage of requiring less time and effort directed toward clinical training and support. For some clinics, based on available resources or the patient population, experienced midlevel providers may be the only feasible option for NP and PA staffing needs.

To prevent unnecessary turnover and set the foundation for a positive employment relationship, facilities hiring experienced NPs and PAs must also set performance expectations and provide a supportive management structure. Consider the following support systems for experienced providers:

- Clinical training—NPs and PAs acquire the majority of clinical skills and knowledge from previous employment. As a result, hiring two midlevel providers with the same number of years' experience does not necessarily translate to a similar level of clinical knowledge. Even experienced midlevel providers may require clinical training.
- Access to resources—Experienced midlevel providers are more comfortable with and capable of making clinical decisions despite a gap in knowledge. Investing in clinical resources as a reference helps NPs and PAs diagnose and treat patients in your facility without referring questions to another provider. Give providers a budget for subscriptions to such materials or provide them in your practice.
- Access to experience— In some settings, experienced NPs and PAs may be capable of and comfortable with practicing autonomously without another provider on site. Providing access by phone or another mode of communication to a more specialized or experienced provider is helpful when questions arise about patient care.
- Feedback—While experienced providers may need little help with day-to-day clinical responsibilities, managerial, personal, and other issues are bound to arise that affect the employer-employee relationship. Avoid mistaking clinical competency as a sign that the provider is satisfied in his or her current position. Maintain a line of open communication by scheduling time for regular feedback.
- Continuing education—Encourage experienced midlevel providers to continue learning new skills. This makes the NP and PA even more valuable in the clinical setting and signals that you are invested in the provider's career and professional growth.

WHEN THINGS GO RIGHT

Hiring midlevel providers may seem like an exhausting undertaking, demanding of your and your staff's time and energy. You may have even received pushback from other physicians or practice administrators who cited the NP and PA learning curve and requirement for support as reasons not to hire an NP or PA.

When implemented effectively, however, providing a support system can be beneficial for all providers and benefits the culture and productivity of your practice as a whole.

A hospital CEO I recently spoke with understands this concept and has a clear vision for using nurse practitioners and physician assistants to create stability and value in the hospital's affiliated clinics and specialty practices.

Rurally located, the hospital has difficulty recruiting and retaining providers. "When a physician quits or retires, we're totally hosed!" he lamented. Patient volumes and financial models don't allow for staffing a larger physician workforce, so the hospital is turning to NPs and PAs.

A nurse practitioner is hired for each physician on staff at the hospital. The NP works in conjunction with the physician practicing in the designated specialty. The physician is responsible for mentoring the nurse practitioner, helping the NP increase clinical knowledge and skills to the level where the nurse practitioner is comfortable working autonomously. This relationship provides several advantages for providers, patients, and the facility.

While patient volumes may not entirely justify a second provider, in this scenario, the cost of employing a nurse practitioner is significantly less than employing a physician. As a result, the facility can afford a second, billing, provider. This decreases wait times for patients, improves customer service, and accommodates increased patient volumes, generating additional revenue for the facility.

For physicians, the relationship means a better work-life balance. Rounding and clinic responsibilities are delegated to nurse practitioners, so the pressure to serve as the sole provider for a subset of patients dissipates, which leads to reduced rates of physician turnover. In the clinic, the physician is able to spend more time with complex patients, making for a more intellectually stimulating practice. Surgeons have more time in the operating room, generating revenue.

Finally, and most important to the chronically stressed hospital CEO, when a physician does leave the hospital, the role can be temporarily filled by the highly trained nurse practitioner. Even if the NP can't take over completely, activity in the department resumes at a baseline capacity. A provider vacancy becomes less critical to the success of the hospital as a whole.

THE MIDLEVEL PROVIDER PAY OFFS

The effort put into recruiting and retaining midlevel providers pays off and manifests itself in the following ways:
1. Increased financial benefits;
2. Increased productivity and efficiency;
3. Improved job satisfaction;
4. Decreased rate of burnout; and
5. Improved practice culture.

Increased financial benefits

As discussed in Chapter 4, employing nurse practitioners and physician assistants confers several financial benefits to a medical practice. A generally accepted metric is that nurse practitioners and physician assistants can treat about 80% of the patients of a physician in the primary care setting. Salaries for these midlevel providers, however, are significantly lower than those of physicians.

According to the U.S. Department of Labor Bureau of Labor Statistics, the mean annual wage in 2015 was $101,260 for nurse practitioners and $99,270 for physician assistants. In contrast, the mean annual wage for family and general physicians weighed in at $192,120. The disparity in salary between midlevel providers and physicians coupled with the ability to treat the majority of the same patients points to significant cost savings by employing NPs and PAs.

Studies also indicate that employing midlevel providers decreases practice overhead compared with exclusively physician employment. A 2004 study, for example, showed practices that use NPs and PAs more extensively in providing care realized lower labor costs per visit than practices making less extensive use of midlevel providers.[1] Estimates for the labor cost savings associated with midlevel providers range from 5% to 9% per primary care visit.

Not only do practices overall realize financial benefits with midlevel provider utilization, physician salaries also see a boost. A 2013 MGMA report, *Physician Compensation and Production Module,* for example, shows that compensation is higher for physicians who employ non-physician providers across all specialties.[2]

Increased productivity and efficiency

The typical patient experience in the outpatient setting begins with being escorted to an exam room, sitting on a noisy paper cover draped over a vinyl exam bed, then having one's vital signs taken. In the majority of cases, a medical assistant rather than a nurse completes these tasks. Employing a nurse to escort patients and take blood pressures often is unnecessary and costly. A lower wage employee can get the job done. When it comes to the provider role, however, most medical practices do the opposite. They employ physicians to perform work that could be done by a nurse practitioner. The result? They are missing out on potential revenue.

Dr. Joseph Guarisco, system chair for emergency medicine at the Ochsner Health System, reports the facility's emergency department has realized significant return on investment by hiring midlevel providers.

The average cost of employing nurse practitioners at the facility is $114,000 annually. This is only 25%–35% the compensation for physicians in the same department. He reports that midlevel providers employed in the emergency department are 80% as productive as their physician counterparts. After adjusting the cost of employing a midlevel provider for productivity, NPs and PAs at the facility result in a 50% savings when it comes to salary.[3]

In nearly all healthcare facilities, whether in the acute hospital setting or in primary care clinics, physicians are doing work that lower cost workers are capable of handling. Delegating this workload to midlevel providers has an immediate positive effect on the facility's bottom line.

Cost savings may be reinvested in the company to help facilities achieve other goals. Savings, for example, give facilities the financial means to bring additional providers on board, decreasing wait times and improving patient satisfaction scores, a metric of increasing importance in today's healthcare environment. Hiring nurse practitioners and physician assistants has the potential to increase profits along with patient volume and satisfaction.

Improved job satisfaction

As mentioned earlier in the chapter, the physicians responsible for training me in the emergency department embarked on a months-long process. The benefit of these physicians' work? A more-than-seven-years (and counting) employment relationship with a nurse practitioner who works almost autonomously unless treating the highest acuity patients in the emergency department.

Traditionally, in the emergency department, physicians lament the constant flow of non-acute patients. ED physicians became doctors to see some action, to treat *sick* patients. Employing a team of highly trained nurse practitioners and physician assistants frees up physicians' time to focus on acute patients. The responsibility for patients with lower acuity problems falls on midlevel providers.

In a healthcare environment where the way physicians practice is increasingly dictated by third-party payers and government organizations, hiring a midlevel provider frees the physician to take back some control of his or her practice by focusing on the cases the physician finds most interesting and those that require the most advanced skills.

Decreased rate of burnout

A former nurse practitioner classmate of mine, Sarah, works for a thriving cardiology group. New to the specialty, it took several months for Sarah to become comfortable treating these patients and to become accustomed to the practice's flow. But, once she did, she became a tremendous asset to the team.

Tired of endless call responsibilities and rounding on weekends, cardiologists in the group began to employ midlevel providers and train them. Now, these NPs and PAs are the first ones to answer calls and assist with weekend rounding on patients. Fewer consultation requests make it through to cardiologists after hours. Time spent rounding is significantly reduced. The group has effectively spread out less-desirable job responsibilities at an affordable cost, creating a better lifestyle for everyone on the team.

Burnout is epidemic among physicians. Surveys consistently show that approximately one in every three physicians is experiencing burnout at any given time.[4] Workload and lack of work-life balance are commonly cited reasons.

Physicians graduate from medical residencies with an acute awareness as to what it looks like to work long hours, spend weekends on call, and function on inadequate sleep. Carrying this work ethic with them as they begin their careers, they quickly find the lifestyle exhausting. A lack of flexibility limits the freedom the physician imagined that a healthcare paycheck would provide. Working odd hours may interfere with personal relationships and a social schedule. As a result, lack of enthusiasm for the medical profession takes root.

Spending more hours at work and working at a faster pace are not sustainable measures to meet the demands of patient care. Adding midlevel medical providers to your practice addresses many factors that lead to physician burnout. Hiring additional healthcare providers may allow physicians to work shorter hours, decrease call responsibilities, and allow for more flexible scheduling. Freeing up time by using midlevel providers allows physicians to spend more time away from work pursuing personal endeavors and relationships. Sure, expanding your team will cost something, but how much are your time and relationships worth?

Improved practice culture

Healthcare is delivered in a complex organizational environment. Healthcare facilities are notoriously behind when it comes to the intentional creation of workplace culture. Coupled, these two realities quickly throw many health systems into a downward spiral that results in turnover and employee and patient dissatisfaction.

Interacting with patients does not always come easily. Healthcare providers may find themselves working with different personalities and individuals apathetic about their own well-being. The need to be "on" day after day, week after week, is wearing, not to mention the fact that dealing with bureaucracy and red tape in an increasingly regulated healthcare system limits providers' ability to work efficiently and effectively. Disillusioned, burned-out providers have little energy left to invest in other staff. Patience wears thin. Frustrations become apparent.

Constructing a positive practice culture starts at the top, with administrators and providers. If your providers aren't happy, the rest of your employees won't be happy either. Both positive and negative attitudes have a trickle-down effect, reaching employees at every level. It's up to you as a leader to choose which will prevail in your practice.

Maintaining a positive outlook is virtually impossible for the overworked, burned-out physician. Unburdening practice leaders with the help of NPs and PAs stops negative cycles and allows for the creation of a positive practice culture.

Improving job satisfaction and decreasing burnout among physicians by utilizing midlevel providers allows physicians to become more effective in leadership roles. Reduced stress, a brighter career outlook, and improved work-life balance have a positive effect on the practice overall. In turn, leadership leads to greater job satisfaction in the organization as a whole.

IN SUMMARY

Implementing simple strategies for training and supporting midlevel providers in your practice leads to financial and lifestyle rewards for those who take the time to do so. Business mogul Richard Branson perhaps summed this idea up the best saying "Train people well enough so they can leave, treat them well enough so they don't want to." You get in what you put out when it comes to employment relationships.

REFERENCES

1. Roblin DW, Howard DH, and Becker ER. (2004). Use of midlevel practitioners to achieve labor cost savings in the primary care practice of an MCO. *Health Services Research.* 39(3):607-626. Retrieved September 23, 2016, from www.ncbi.nlm.nih.gov/pmc/articles/PMC1361027/.
2. Medical Group Management Association. *NPP Utilization in the Future of U.S. Healthcare.* Englewood, CO: MGMA; 2013. Retrieved September 24, 2016, from http://online.mgma.org/npp-report-download.
3. Guarisco J, MD. Mid-Level Providers – Who they are, what they do, and why they're changing emergency medicine. *EP Monthly.* 2014. Retrieved September 12, 2016, from http://epmonthly.com/article/mid-level-providers-who-they-are-what-they-do-and-why-they-re-changing-emergency-medicine.
4. Shanafelt TD, MD. (2009). Enhancing meaning in work: A prescription for preventing physician burnout and promoting patient-centered care. *JAMA.* 302(12):1338-1340.

CHAPTER 6

Best Midlevel Provider Hiring Practices

Compensation, expectation, and transparency

People leave their bosses, not their jobs. A recent Gallup study of more than 7,200 employees found that more than 50% have left a job to get away from a manager.[1] So, how do employees decide if their bosses are "bad" or "good"?

One of the most significant factors identified in the study was reliable and meaningful communication, especially regarding job expectations and responsibilities. Dissatisfied workers felt that they were given little guidance for understanding what was expected of them. According to the poll, just 12% of employees feel that their bosses help set work priorities and give clear expectations. That 12% are much happier at work than those who rank their bosses lower on these measures. Gallup's report notes that "Clarity of expectations is perhaps the most basic of employee needs and is vital to performance."

While "clarity of expectations" seems easy to communicate given that healthcare providers are educated to function within a specific role, my conversations with nurse practitioners, physician assistants, and medical practices around the country indicate there is significant room for improvement when it comes to such conversations.

I recently spoke with a nurse practitioner, Jennifer, who felt like she was failing in her role. Frustrated and near tears, she expressed disappointment that her employer was not more supportive. As a recent graduate, she had clinical questions, but had difficulty getting answers from colleagues. She suspected her boss was disappointed in her performance since she personally felt like she was failing in her role. Jennifer was poised to quit her job.

The primary care practice where Jennifer worked was a client of my company, so I called the physician CEO to get feedback on her performance. "We love Jennifer," I was surprised to hear him say. "She has a lot to learn, but her patients regularly stop by the reception desk as they leave to share how much they enjoyed having her as their provider." He continued, "Patient experience is the most important thing to me. I can teach clinical efficiency, but I need providers who make patients want to come back to see us."

The physician measured success of midlevel providers based on patient satisfaction. The nurse practitioner was measuring her own success based on patient volume and clinical skill set. The lack of communication as to what made her a valuable provider was nearly a costly misunderstanding.

61

The frustration and dissatisfaction Jennifer felt was quickly cleared up after just a few conversations. Had expectations not been clarified, she may have quit her position, leaving the practice with a costly vacancy and the hassle of finding a new provider to fill the role.

Similar to job responsibilities and expectations, practices must also clearly outline compensation for midlevel providers, as dissatisfaction or disputes related to pay are equally as likely to result in a damaged employment relationship between the employer and midlevel provider.

Compensation conflicts are prevalent in healthcare. Reimbursement models followed by insurance companies and government entities are complex. So, employer compensation models built on productivity seem anything but transparent to the provider.

Nurse practitioners and physician assistants are wary of the promise of bonuses and an RVU-based paycheck, as the criteria for receiving such compensation is often vaguely laid out or based on financial data to which the provider does not have access. Quickly, such models lead to distrust on by the midlevel provider as illustrated in the scenario with my first employer discussed in Chapter 1 of this book.

Although the process of reimbursement for healthcare services by third-party payers is complex, employers must shield providers from these bureaucratic systems by outlining clear compensation structures. This serves to reinforce the role and expectations of the provider and sets the foundation for transparency and trust in the employment relationship. It clearly shows NPs and PAs what is required of them to earn more money.

By clearly outlining the role, expectations, and responsibilities of midlevel providers in your practice, you avoid the major pitfalls that most commonly result in provider dissatisfaction and strained employment relationships.

OUTLINING JOB RESPONSIBILITIES AND COMPENSATION

Dissatisfaction with employment among nurse practitioners and physician assistants almost always begins with lack of clarity around compensation and/or job expectations. My first employment contract as an NP specified that I could be awarded a quarterly productivity bonus. The method by which the bonus would be calculated, however, was nebulous. Hard-working providers naturally assumed they would be awarded a bonus. However, bonus checks never arrived in our mailboxes. So, turnover among midlevel providers in the practice was common.

RVU-based productivity compensation models have similar drawbacks. While employers use these compensation structures to incentivize hard work, they are anything but transparent. They reinforce the frustrations associated with a bureaucratic healthcare system rather than allowing the employees to think positively about their job. They trap employers into inefficient staffing systems, as pay is based primarily on the number of patients the provider sees and the quantity of services provided, rather than on growth of the practice through effective teamwork and quality customer service.

Finally, the lack of transparency inherent in these compensation models erodes the midlevel providers' trust in the employer and mars the employment relationship.

Fortunately, there is a better way to reward hard-working providers. Compensation structures must be written and clearly presented in conjunction with job responsibilities. As job responsibilities and clinical competency increase, so should compensation.

Not only is a written compensation document essential for a satisfying employment relationship built on trust, it also motivates midlevel providers to advance their clinical skills and take on additional responsibilities in the practice. It ensures that conversations about employment expectations occur, so the practice does not fall victim to the common managerial mistakes outlined in the Gallup survey mentioned earlier.

The Compensation Levels Document

Set the standard for compensation of midlevel providers in your practice by creating a compensation levels document. This document clearly outlines pay for midlevel providers as it relates to their essential responsibilities and the expectations for NPs and PAs in your practice. It indicates the NP's or PA's salary at the level where the provider meets basic expectations; by taking on additional responsibility and skills, the midlevel provider earns more, arriving at the next pay level.

The compensation levels document takes three things into account to determine salary:

1. Years of experience;
2. Clinical scope of practice; and
3. Professional skill level.

As you work to create levels of responsibility and corresponding compensation, think deliberately about where dividing lines for scope of responsibility and skills should lie. Make these dividing lines as clear as possible to avoid confusion or controversy. Ideally, you should have between five and seven levels of compensation for midlevel providers in your practice. Each level outlines the responsibilities, skills, or expectations required to reach the indicated salary.

To help create your scopes of responsibility for each level, start by imagining that you have a large practice with 20 midlevel providers of varying ability. What would be the most helpful way to segment them? You could have less-experienced providers treat low acuity patients. Or, you may assign fewer patients to less-experienced providers. Alternately, you may rely on providers to build their own patient panels, segregating them by the number of patients on their panel. The most-experienced midlevel providers may serve in managerial roles, responsible for managing a subset of other providers. If you are in an academic setting, you may financially reward providers for research or participation in clinical trials through the various levels in your compensation document.

Next, determine the specific responsibilities that should be identified in each level as a measure to determine providers' salary. Think about what is most important to you and your practice and include these items in your various scopes of responsibility. Is there something that recurrently annoys you in your role as an overseeing physician? If so, include this behavior in the compensation levels document.

For example, does answering midlevel providers' clinical questions that may be easily answered by looking a medical reference book take valuable time away from your own work? Include something along the lines of "Uses clinical resources as the first line for finding information and answers to questions" as a requirement to move up from the lowest rung on the compensation ladder.

Some categories you may want to consider as part of your scope of responsibility for midlevel providers include:
- Patient volume;
- Patient satisfaction;
- Procedural skills;
- Clinical support required;
- Adherence to and/or knowledge of systems, processes, and resources (e.g., EMR, CMS guidelines);
- Non-clinical responsibilities (e.g., marketing, management);
- Professionalism;
- Administrative responsibilities; and/or
- Involvement in research or education projects.

Motivate nurse practitioners and physician assistants by outlining exactly what it takes to be an exceptional midlevel provider in your practice and by paying accordingly. Your levels document will make these steps toward excellence transparent for your team so that NPs and PAs understand what it takes to improve and how to prioritize these responsibilities.

As you brainstorm to create your own levels document, think about how you might include these measures in your assessment:

Patient volume
Nurse practitioners and physician assistants with time management skills that allow for higher patient volume naturally generate more revenue and should be compensated accordingly. You may develop a patient volume expectation for each level in your compensation structure.

For example, in the primary care setting, the lowest level of compensation may specify that the nurse practitioner "Completes an average of 1.5 established patient appointments per hour." Alternately or additionally, you may wish to specify the number of patients the provider maintains as part of his or her patient panel and link this to level of compensation.

Patient satisfaction

As patient satisfaction becomes increasingly tied to reimbursement, you may wish to link customer satisfaction with provider pay. Verbiage such as "Receives fewer than three patient complaints per six-month period," "Receives at least two positive comment cards per month," "Maintains an average patient satisfaction rating of 4 on a 5-point scale," or simply "Regularly receives positive feedback from patients" may be outlined in your compensation levels document.

Clinical skill set

Most nurse practitioners and physician assistants must learn to perform procedures skillfully, along with attaining additional clinical knowledge as part of employment. Procedural skills are not commonly mastered as part of most schools' curricula. If performing certain procedures is important to a provider's efficacy in your practice, compensate accordingly. Outline which procedures the provider must be able to perform, and to what degree, at each level in the compensation document.

If there are any professional designations or supplemental degrees that are relevant to your specialty or the level of responsibility you would like midlevel providers to reach, you may also wish to include these in the compensation levels document.

Required support

Less-experienced providers require more support in the day-to-day clinical environment. Reward increased autonomy by linking independent practice and improved clinical competency to pay. For example, "Diagnoses and treats clinically complex patients autonomously" may be included at the highest level of compensation. "Requires direct or frequent involvement from physician to treat clinically complex patients" may be at the bottom rung of the compensation chart.

You may even choose to be more specific, stating something along the lines of, "When asking a question about a patient, leads with what the provider thinks is the problem or diagnosis and, more often than not, the supporting physician agrees" or "Upon diagnosing a patient, knows the next steps in treatment."

Systems, processes, and resources

Adhering to an increasing number of practice guidelines dictated by entities like CMS, JHACO, and large hospital systems themselves can be difficult and can contribute to job dissatisfaction. Turn the tables and increase your practice's compliance with such measures, as well as job satisfaction, by rewarding providers who comply with required guidelines.

For example, if providers are hesitant to use certain features of your facility's EMR system, include "Follows practice standards for EMR usage on at least 90% of patient charts" on higher levels of your compensation document. Or, you may include specific items like "Adheres to guidelines for management of sepsis in at least 85% of patients" if this is relevant to your practice.

Set your standards to be specific and measurable to avoid questions about whether the expectation has been met.

Non-clinical responsibilities

Brian, a physician assistant friend of mine working at an academic center, recently recounted with humor some surprises he encountered in his new position. One day, during his first month at the facility, the department's marketing manager asked that he accompany her on an all-day excursion around the city to promote the practice.

Brian, one orthopedic surgeon, and the chatty marketing manager piled into her car and traveled to clinics around the region promoting the facility's orthopedic services in hopes of gaining referrals.

"I thought I was going to be assisting with surgery," Brain commented, "but forget billable hours, the surgeon and I spent all day shaking hands."

Unanticipated workplace activities such as this marketing excursion kept Brian away from doing what he loved: working in the operating room and assisting surgeons. The perceived inefficiency of such responsibilities eventually led him to dread his job. These expectations had not been made clear when he accepted the position and weren't associated with any perceived benefit on Brian's part.

Do you expect midlevel providers to engage in marketing efforts to help build their patient panel and promote the practice? Or, would you like capable providers to take on managerial responsibilities? If you work in an academic facility, do you expect nurse practitioners and physician assistants to publish, collect data, or otherwise participate in research?

Outline these items in the compensation levels document. This motivates providers to engage in these responsibilities and shows what it takes outside of patient care to be successful in your practice.

Professionalism

Midlevel providers represent your practice in the way they consult with or refer to other providers and practices as well their interactions with patients. Their attitudes significantly influence workplace culture as they are looked upon by staff as leaders. Consider including aspects of professional behavior as part of midlevel providers' scope of responsibility. "Maintains a good working relationship with staff" or "speaks with poise and confidence to patients and coworkers," for example, may be important to the culture of your practice.

Structuring Compensation

Carefully consider the payment structure for midlevel providers in your practice. The decision between offering salaried, hourly, of productivity-based wages is not inconsequential. Which model will best reinforce your effort for transparency?

Base Compensation

Nurse practitioners and physician assistants may be paid on an hourly, salaried, or productivity basis. Some employers use a combination of two structures. Base salary or hourly wages should specifically be named in the compensation document.

Salaried compensation leads to the healthiest employment relationships. This structure avoids nit-picking about lunch breaks and other petty time issues. It is the most transparent compensation model and therefore fosters a greater element of trust between the employer and provider.

Hourly compensation is also straightforward, with a few caveats. Specify the number of hours the nurse practitioner or physician assistant will be expected to work each week in the employment agreement. If you plan to reduce the provider's hours in the event patient volume decreases, you must be clear about your plan in the hiring process or the employment relationship will be severely damaged. Avoid reducing or adding to a provider's agreed-upon number of hours, even if allowable within the employment contract, as this creates an element of distrust and dissatisfaction on part of the provider.

Compensating midlevel providers based on productivity is not advisable. This structure is difficult, if not impossible for the provider to track and consistently leaves doubt in the provider's mind as whether their paycheck is fair or even correct. It creates a competitive rather than collaborative workplace and limits your options for creative staffing solutions. A clearly outlined compensation levels document motivates providers to be productive while shielding them from the dissatisfaction-causing complexities of our healthcare system. If you must pay providers on a productivity-based model, clearly document how pay will be calculated and share this in a written document as part of the hiring process.

Bonuses and/or Commissions

Ideally, practices should stick to a flat salary or hourly compensation model without bonuses. The "bonus" comes as the provider increases scope of responsibility and skill in the practice, as outlined in your compensation levels document.

If you do choose to incentivize midlevel providers with bonuses, just as with base compensation, bonuses should be transparently outlined in the document. Describe when and how these will be paid, as well as the amount. Consider having a separate document that details the bonus or commission structures to compliment the compensation document.

Creating Your Own Compensation Levels Document

Creating your own compensation levels document requires an initial investment of time and thought. This process is well worth the effort as it saves infinitely more time on the back end by avoiding unnecessary compensation disputes and by encouraging performance and setting priorities that align with those of the practice.

Follow these steps to create your own compensation levels document. Use the sample compensation levels document included at the end of this chapter as a guide.

Step 1

Think about everything that frustrates or annoys you about your current and past experiences employing midlevel providers. In a cathartic brainstorm, write it down! Consider including these items as actions midlevel providers must consistently display to move from the lowest compensation level to the next step up.

Step 2

Look through the list of components suggested earlier in this chapter. List responsibilities and/or characteristics of midlevel providers that are important to you in each category. Identify those that are the most important.

Step 3

Create five to seven different levels for both Clinical Scope of Practice and Professional Skill. Place the items from your previous lists under each level based on the skill required to carry out the responsibility. Refine the requirements for each level so that the dividing lines between scopes of responsibility are as clear as possible.

Step 4

Assign a salary or hourly rate to each level. This is the dollar amount the NP or PA can expect to earn by performing to the standards specified in each level. You may use advanced practice provider compensation data from your area or determine pay based on the compensation of providers currently employed by your practice.

Ideally, the compensation levels document will not change significantly over time. This is a stable structure that midlevel providers can rely on to outline expectations for performance and metrics for achievement.

A transparent, multi-level compensation structure allows midlevel providers to determine how success will be measured in their role. It gives direction, showing providers where to focus their time and energy. Implementing a compensation levels document builds a foundation of trust on which the employment relationship is built, leading to open, cooperative conversations about pay.

FINDING THE RIGHT MIDLEVEL PROVIDER FOR THE JOB

My father-in-law is an accomplished businessman who worked for The Dow Chemical Company, then Eli Lilly, over the course of his career. His managerial and administrative roles in these companies required that he frequently interview candidates to fill open positions. As his children and their friends began to seek post-college employment, he trained them to interview for competitive positions using a system he had developed.

Even before I became a nurse practitioner, my dream had always been to work in an emergency department. Unable to get so much as a call back from area hospitals as a new graduate, I kicked off my career in primary care and urgent care. So, after two years, when I finally landed an interview at a local hospital for an emergency department position, I sought my father-in-law's help preparing for the big day.

I sat for hours in his office preparing through mock interview scenarios and interview coaching. As part of my interview training, I wrote outlines reminding myself about challenges I had overcome and leadership scenarios where I had effectively taken charge. I even practiced walking through the door and greeting my interviewer with a firm handshake. While I may not have had the clinical experience required for the job in the ED, I was ready to prove that I could learn to do so.

On the day of my interview, I ironed my rarely worn black slacks and blazer. I paired them with conservative black heels and a string of tasteful pearls. I carefully placed a few copies of my resume, printed on thick, quality paper, into a newly purchased black folio and marched out the door.

When I arrived at the hospital, I met the director of the department and was given a brief tour. Arriving back at the director's office, I handed him my resume and we chatted for a minute or two. Then, to my astonishment, he offered me the job. There were no "What are your biggest strengths and weaknesses?" questions or "Tell me about a time when…" requests. To my knowledge, he didn't even contact my references. Just a tour and a job offer.

Perhaps I shouldn't have been surprised by the brevity and simplicity of the interview. Interviews for my prior positions in the primary care practice and urgent care clinic had gone similarly. In fact, during my eight years, three full-time jobs, and few PRN positions I've held throughout my nurse practitioner career, I've never had what I would consider a "real" interview. My interviews for nurse practitioner jobs have consisted of a tour of the practice and a rundown of how things function in the facility, followed by some version of "we pay X dollars per hour, the job's yours if you want it."

I wish I could say that this has been my experience because I am a genius diagnostician or make a superb first impression. But, I don't think this is the case. Many nurse practitioners whom I send out to interview with healthcare facilities as part of my company's programs email back similarly confused. "The interview wasn't really much of an interview because the medical director didn't really ask me any questions. It didn't feel like an interview. I am not sure where we go from here. Will they contact me if they are interested?" emailed a nurse practitioner last year after her interview with a hospital that is part of a major health system. Her interviewer apparently asked little about her, making her unsure about the possibility of future employment—not to mention she wasn't offered any guidance about next steps in the process. The medical director, however, had informed me that the interview went wonderfully and that this nurse practitioner was the facility's top candidate for the position.

If you want to utilize nurse practitioners and physician assistants effectively in your practice, you're going to need to find the right person for the job. And, you aren't going to find the right person without asking questions. Identifying a midlevel provider who is a culture fit for your practice requires an effective, systematized interview strategy.

Know What You're Looking For

Many medical practices mistakenly assume that because the role of healthcare providers in a specific setting remains relatively consistent across employers, they simply must find a candidate for the job who is certified, licensed, and capable of performing the designated skill set. While this may partially be the case, there are a number of problems with this approach.

First, it is difficult to assess clinical skills in the interview setting. You can't ask job applicants to demonstrate on patients. Your best bet when it comes to clinical competency is to rely on candidate self-assessment, references, and the amount of prior experience. However, this doesn't always translate into performing the required clinical skills efficiently and proficiently.

Second, it is essential to identify a provider who fits your practice culture. The new member on your team must work well with existing employees within the practice environment. If your practice values volume, you'll need a hard-working, efficient provider who can achieve this outcome. If your practice is more relational and emphasizes patient experience, you'll need a midlevel provider capable of delivering this style of care.

The importance of identifying a midlevel provider who fits your practice culture cannot be overstated. It's easier to teach a provider who works well with your existing team and is motivated to learn, than one with the required clinical skills who isn't a natural fit for the group. Think critically about the characteristics of the provider you're looking for before you start the interview process. Don't fall into the trap of hiring the wrong person for the job simply because you need to fill the position or because the individual looks good on paper.

Screening Resumes

The number of resumes you can expect to receive for a midlevel provider opening varies widely. In a rural, medically underserved community, you may be crossing your fingers and praying to receive one partially qualified applicant. Major health systems or large academic health centers may receive hundreds of applicants for a single position. Regardless of the camp you fall into, the basic principles are the same when it comes to sorting through resumes.

Resumes share notoriously little information about a candidate. So, they are more useful for identifying negatives. Resumes with sloppy formatting, poor grammar, and multiple misspellings, for example, absolutely must be screened out, no matter how desperate you are to hire for the position. If the provider didn't take the time to format the resume or proofread the document, you can imagine how his or her patient charts will hold up if ever called into question by a court of law.

Develop a set of objective measures by which you score resumes. This scoring system can also help you decide in which order to interview candidates. You may choose to look at some of the following measures:

- Background—While clinical experience is certainly worth considering, applicants with backgrounds in other professional areas also bring valuable perspective to your practice. A former human resources manager turned nurse practitioner, for example, may be helpful when it comes to hiring and making other managerial decisions in the future. A former IT professional may be invaluable when the practice implements a new EHR system.
- Accomplishments—Your applicant may not have attended an Ivy League graduate program, but does he or she have other impressive accomplishments listed on the resume? Military experience, for example, shows evidence of hard work and dedication. Such accomplishments, even if not clinically related, should be weighted highly in the resume screening process.
- Organizational Interest—Does it appear that the applicant has submitted hundreds of resumes to various practices across the country on websites like CareerBuilder? Or, was the resume submitted with a well-written cover letter based on interest specifically in your practice? Applicants who submit resumes based on some sort of selection criteria and with a specific interest in your practice are more worth your time.
- Paperwork—The certification of the provider must match up with the patient population you're hiring to treat. An adult-gerontology nurse practitioner, for example, may not be the best fit for a family practice, as this NP won't be able to see kids. Make sure the qualifications listed on the resume logistically line up with the position you're trying to fill.

Remember, these are simply the criteria by which you're deciding whether to toss the resume in the paper shredder or to stick it under the paperweight on your desk for a call back. These are not the criteria by which you're hiring. Resumes that you deem worthy make it to the next step in the process: the phone interview.

The Phone Interview

Even if you receive a resume from a candidate who lives two miles away from your practice, you'll want to start the interview process with a phone interview. This serves as a screening process, saves time and money, and allows you to hone in on some important qualities of the candidate before meeting in person. It allows you to talk with candidates who look good on paper, screening out those who don't live up to their paper persona in conversation.

Try breaking your phone screen into three parts:

1. Candidate introduces him/herself (10 minutes);
2. Interviewer introduces him/herself (10 minutes); and
3. Q&A: Candidate asks questions (10 minutes).

Start the call by letting the candidates know how the interview will be structured. While there is a structure to your call, allow conversation to flow. If the candidates struggle with spending more than a few minutes talking about themselves, ask questions about what they have told you so far or that appear on their resumes. You might ask, for example, why the candidate decided to become a nurse practitioner, or how he/she selected a graduate program.

As you listen and talk, assess the candidates' qualities. Do they speak with poise? Do they seem intelligent? Is there evidence that they have done due diligence and researched your practice before the call? Red flags such as a failure to do one's homework when it comes to learning about your practice, or speaking in a manner you wouldn't feel comfortable putting in front of patients in your practice, allows you to eliminate unqualified applicants.

If your candidate seems to have promise, offer an in-person interview at the end of the call. Avoid making hiring decisions until you have met the individual and conducted a formal in-person interview.

The In-Person Interview

The final stage of the hiring process is the in-person interview. You should have an idea as to your candidate's qualifications and fit for the practice by this stage, but keep an open mind as you enter the face-to-face interview. You want to be able to identify red flags, and green flags as well, throughout the course of your interaction.

Ideally, the candidate will interview in a similar manner with multiple individuals in your practice. At the very least, the candidate should also interview with one individual who would work alongside the candidate in the clinical setting—another physician, nurse practitioner, or physician assistant. Clinicians will have different takeaways from an interview than the HR department or administrators and vice versa. By having the candidate interview with multiple parties, you get a well-rounded view of the provider and, most importantly, the approval of the candidate's future colleagues for the new addition.

Don't forget that in the interview process, the candidate is interviewing you as an employer as well. It is important that the interaction is mutually beneficial and that the candidate comes away with a sense of the culture of your practice. As the one conducting the interview, it is your responsibility to make sure the candidate understands the responsibilities of the job as well as who he or she will be working with.

Good candidates are likely looking at a number of different employment options, so show what distinguishes your practice from others. Setting the tone for transparency when it comes to job expectations and responsibilities starts early, and you should share this in the interview process. It will be part of what helps you stand out from other employment options the candidate might have.

Starting the Interview

To start the in-person interview, take five minutes or so to chat with the candidate. This creates a relaxed, conversational atmosphere. It ensures that you see the "real" candidate for the job. Ask where the candidate is from or what he/she likes to do for fun. Show interest and let the conversation flow naturally.

Begin the focused part of the interview by asking something along the lines of, "To get started, why don't you tell me about your understanding of this position." This allows you to clear up any misconceptions of the job and describe it in more detail. You will also get an idea as to how well the candidate prepared for the interview by researching your practice in advance.

Continuing the Interview

Have the candidate's resume handy and ask him/her to walk you through the resume. Start with college, and continue with a recap of each job held thereafter. While this may seem redundant, given that the information has already been presented to you in writing, it can reveal several important characteristics of the candidate. Joel Spolsky, CEO of Stack Overflow, suggests paying attention to three particular aspects of the candidate:[2]

1. Whether he/she is driven;
2. Whether he/she has passion; and
3. How he/she makes decisions.

While these items may not correlate directly with the candidate's current skill set, they do reveal motivation to learn and become an effective, efficient team player. They also show you how the candidate might apply clinical knowledge.

Consider asking questions similar the following to hone in on these aspects.

1. How have you made major life decisions?
   - Why did you pick that school?
   - How did you decide on that major?
   - How did you decide to take/leave that job?
2. What were some of your achievements at that job?
3. What are some examples of mistakes you've made? How would you have done things differently now?
4. What were some of your favorite parts of that position?
5. What were some of the challenges with each job?
6. What were you hired to do in each job?
7. What would your boss say about you?
8. Who were the people you worked most closely with? How would they describe you?

Follow your Q&A of the candidate by giving him/her some time to ask his/her own questions. If you think this is a candidate you want to move forward with, you may also want to take time at this point to show him/her around the clinical area where he/she would be working and introduce him/her to potential coworkers.

Ending the Interview

If you haven't ruled out the candidate, end the interview by asking permission to check his/her references. Ask if there is anyone your candidate would like you *not* to contact, such as the candidate's current employer. You may also wish to ask the candidate to connect you via email with the references he/she suggests you contact.

Making a Decision

Throughout the interview conversation, you will notice red flags—a warning the candidate may not be the right hire—or green flags—assurance the candidate is a fit for the position. Note that red flags and green flags aren't set in stone. While being late to an interview is certainly a red flag, calling in advance to explain that he/she is stuck in traffic may be more of a green flag. Another example might be that the candidate's ability to talk about prior experiences could be a green flag, however, talking far too much and dominating the conversation is a red flag.

Red flags might include:

1. Being late or unprepared for the interview. The candidate should bring a resume and be familiar with the details of the position and your practice, especially those that are readily available online or that were discussed in the phone screen.
2. Complaints about previous employers. A candidate who complains about a previous employer suggests that he/she blames others in the face of challenge. Ideally, the culture of your practice is not one in which complaining is a match.
3. Vague answers as to why the candidate left previous employers. Litigation or disputes with former employers are a major red flag. In some cases, vague answers can mean the candidate is trying to be respectful. If this is the case, the candidate will not give the same reason for each job he/she left.
4. Lack of appropriate references. Candidates who list personal friends as references and who cannot name a supervisor he/she has had within the last five years as a reference likely has a reason. Proceed with caution. Make sure the candidate provides a reference from at least one individual who has supervised the candidate in the clinical setting.
5. Inconsistencies or discomfort around a particular topic. If the candidate becomes visibly uncomfortable when you ask about a job he/she has held, for example, this suggests something is suspicious. The candidate may be covering up a negative experience or lying on his/her resume.
6. The candidate does not have any questions at the end of the interview. If a candidate has been paying attention and engaged during the interview process, he/she should naturally have at least a few questions about the job or the practice. Asking only questions centered around compensation and benefits is also a bad sign, as this can mean a paycheck is the only reason the candidate is considering the job. Many candidates know they will be expected to ask questions and prepare them in advance, which is a good sign. If the candidate lets you know that he/she had questions prepared but these have been covered over the course of the interview, this should not be seen as a red flag.

On the flip side, green flags are signs that the midlevel provider is likely a good fit for the position. Green flags might include:

You have a good conversation with the applicant during the icebreaker portion of the interview. The candidate relaxes and naturally keeps up with the flow of the conversation throughout the interview. Use caution here, as you do want to maintain objectivity. If you like the applicant as a person based on your conversation, it can be difficult to maintain a balanced view of him/her as an applicant.

The provider came prepared with copies of his/her resume and a list of questions to ask during the interview. And, the questions the candidate asks are intelligent and insightful. A list of questions that could have been answered with a quick glance at your practice's website may be a red flag because they indicate lack of preparation.

The candidate presents a balanced picture of him/herself. While the candidate appropriately touts accomplishments, achievements, or rave recommendations, he/she is also able to discuss areas of weakness.

A candidate may reveal something about his or her personal circumstances that might affect his/her employment. Appreciate this level of honesty, as it allows you to accurately assess the provider's fit for the position. Even if these circumstances may be prohibitive now, there is a chance you will be able to hire the prospect later, provided the interview goes well.

Checking References

Recently, I spoke with an applicant to Midlevels for the Medically Underserved, my company's residency-like program for nurse practitioners. Throughout the phone interview, the applicant's pet canary squawked loudly. To me, this was an off-putting professional snafu. However, I didn't feel I could decline the applicant a spot in the program based on this alone, as she was otherwise qualified on paper. Then, the applicant's references arrived in our mailbox. Both references checked the spot for "Average" in the professionalism category on the reference form. Most of our applicants receive "Excellent" ratings across the board. So, this low rating caught my eye, affirming my initial impression. Ultimately, we declined to give the applicant a spot in the program.

Over the course of the next few months, the applicant continued to interact with our company's staff, harassing them over calls and unprofessional emails about the rejection decision. The reference saved us from matching her with a practice who would have undoubtedly been dissatisfied with her level of professionalism.

I've personally talked with hundreds of applicants to this program. While these interview conversations certainly reveal a lot about our applicants, the compliment of a reference to supplement the interview is a powerful combination.

Some applicants may list friends as references, calling into question their workplace abilities or, at very least, their professionalism. Others list references who have directly observed the applicant in the clinical setting who may even take the time to write or call our company to advocate for the applicant's acceptance based on stellar performance. This, of course, speaks volumes and assures we can have confidence sending the nurse practitioner out to work for a partnering facility with our company's name behind them.

While keeping up with references for each applicant isn't always easy, experience shows us it's one of the most important pieces of our interview process.

Reference checks are far too often neglected by healthcare employers. Desperation to fill a provider position may lead employers to cut corners. Or, the mistaken belief that a provider's level of success depends solely on clinical decision-making ability deems them unnecessary.

Checking references is a must before bringing on a new provider. Even if these individuals share very little information about the prospect, simply looking at the individuals the provider lists as potential contacts is helpful. A provider who cannot name any qualified professional references should be a major red flag.

A background check is never a substitute for a reference check. There are plenty of providers out there with clean professional and criminal records who are terrible to work with. Taking the time to talk with multiple references can save you the even more time-consuming pain of hiring the wrong person for the job.

When you call to speak with a candidate's reference, consider structuring the call in the following manner to get as much information as possible without overstepping any boundaries.

1. Introduce yourself, thank the individual for taking the time to talk with you.
2. Ask some or all of the following questions:
   - "In what context have you worked with the candidate and for how long?"
   - "Can you describe the candidate's general responsibilities?"
   - "What were the standards of successful performance in the candidate's role? How did he/she measure up to these standards?"
   - "What would you say are his/her strengths and weaknesses in the clinical setting?"
   - "Would you work with him/her again?"
   - "How would his/her coworkers and/or patients describe him/her?"
3. Thank the reference for their time and wrap up the conversation.

In addition to speaking with at least two references, you must also do your own research on the applicant. Look him/her up on LinkedIn and Facebook. What do you find? Is the candidate's public representation of him/herself something you would feel comfortable with your practice's customers seeing?

In doing your own background research, you might also find out that your professional circles overlap. If you have connections in common, reach out to common contacts. These connections may not be individuals who have observed the provider directly in the workplace, but can still speak to his/her character and accomplishments. Keep in mind the candidate's requests as to who you not contact, such as a current employer. Never check a reference without the candidate's consent and avoid asking for any information that could be used to discriminate against the candidate. Stick to questions about the individual's ability to perform functions relevant to the job.

When you speak with individuals you and the candidate know in common, you are looking for information that helps you decide if the candidate is a good fit for your practice's culture. Consider using the following conversation format when contacting a personal reference:

1. "It looks like you went to school with [the Candidate], is that accurate?"
2. "How did you two meet?"
3. "How long have you known each other?"
4. "Have you been in touch since that time?"
5. "How would his/her peers/coworkers/superiors describe him/her?"
6. "What were some of his/her favorite things to do at [company]? What were some of the things that [the Candidate] didn't enjoy doing?"

Lastly, and most importantly, ask "Who else do you know that I should speak with about [the Candidate]?" Some people may not be willing to share openly about a candidate, but they are willing to connect you with someone who will.

BRINGING THE PROCESS TOGETHER

Overall, clarity and transparency when it comes to the roles and responsibilities of midlevel providers in your practice is essential to job satisfaction and longevity of providers in your practice. Creating a compensation levels document allows you to outline these roles and responsibilities, as well as assign appropriate compensation to match. This document makes it clear to nurse practitioners and physician assistants what success looks like in your practice. It outlines the financial incentive for achievement and is the first step in fostering a healthy employment relationship.

Even with transparency around compensation and expectations, it remains essential to identify the right providers for your practice. Establishing a system for interviewing midlevel providers, vetting their qualifications, and exploring their cultural fit for your workplace pays off. By focusing time and energy on the front end of the hiring process, you ensure that your practice brings on providers who will thrive given the responsibilities encompassed by their role.

REFERENCES

1. Weber L. What do workers want from the boss? *The Wall Street Journal*. April 2, 2015. Retrieved August 10, 2017, from https://blogs.wsj.com/atwork/2015/04/02/what-do-workers-want-from-the-boss/?mod=e2tw.
2. Spolsky J. The guerrilla guide to interviewing (version 3.0). Available at www.joelonsoftware.com/2006/10/25/the-guerrilla-guide-to-interviewing-version-30. October 25, 2006. Accessed March 1, 2017.

SAMPLE COMPENSATION LEVELS DOCUMENT

Providers are central to the success of [Organization Name]. The organization has spent a lot of time thinking about the clinical scope of the responsibility of each of these providers, as well as what professional skills are important for that role. Finally, the company has also evaluated the value that more experience provides our patients and organization.

[Organization Name] uses those three considerations in calculating compensation levels. The chart below gives a general overview of each consideration, and the pages that follow give detail for each category of roles.

Consideration	Description
Clinical Scope	1. What are the result-getting activities of your role? 2. How developed is your clinical skill set? How efficiently do you use these skills in practice? 3. What level of autonomy have you achieved in clinical practice? 4. Are you able to proficiently perform the procedures essential to your role as a provider?
Professionalism	1. Are you effective working with [Organization Name]'s systems and processes? 2. Have you incorporated [Organization Name]'s norms into your own work? 3. Are you able to inspire confidence when working with patients? When working with partnering providers and facilities?
Experience	1. Years working at [Organization Name] count. 2. Years working elsewhere in a midlevel provider role of the same or similar specialty count. 3. Years working in the midlevel provider role in a different specialty may count. 4. Up to [Number] of years working in a related healthcare role, such as nursing, may count. 5. Years working in non-patient facing roles or in other industries do not count.

How to Use the Levels Compensation Document:

Determine level of 'Clinical Scope of Practice' by comparing the midlevel provider's performance and skills to the requirements of each level outlined in the chart.

Determine level of 'Professional Skills' by comparing the midlevel provider's performance and skills to the requirements of each level outlined in the chart.

Take the average of the numerical level for 'Clinical Scope of Practice' and 'Professional Skills' and find this number at the top of the grid.

Using the grid, identify the intersection of the provider's years of experience and the numerical average of scope/professionalism. Use the resulting number in the grid to determine the provider's salary from the salary chart.

Level	1	2	3	4	5	6	7	8	9
Salary	$80,000	$87,500	$95,000	$102,500	$110,000	$117,500	$125,000	$130,000	$135,000

Compensation for 7+ will be based on continuing to inspire the trust of [Organization Name]'s patients — and maintain and grow the relationship with them.

Experience	Average of Scope/Professional Skills						
	1	2	3	4	5	6	7
0-1 years	1	1	1	1	1	1	1
2-3 years	1	2	3	4	5	6	7
4-5 years	2	2	3	4	5	6	7
6-8 years	2	2	3	4	5	6	7
9-11 years	2	3	4	5	6	7	8
12-15 years	3	3	4	5	6	7	8
16-19 years	3	3	4	5	6	7	8
20+ years	3	4	5	6	7	8	9

CLINICAL SCOPE OF PRACTICE

Scope Detail	Description
1	1. Averages [X] patient encounters per hour. 2. Requires direct or indirect involvement from physician to treat more than 50% of patients. 3. Still regularly asks others for information/instruction before using outside resources. 4. Requires oversight with procedures.
2	1. Averages [X] patient encounters per hour. 2. Requires direct or indirect involvement from physician to treat less than 50% of patients. 3. When asking a question about a patient, leads with what the provider thinks is the problem or diagnosis. Consults resources before asking others for instruction. 4. Requires occasional oversight with procedures.
3	1. Averages [X] patient encounters per hour. 2. Requires only occasional involvement from physician to diagnose, make treatment decisions. 3. Proficient in performing basic procedures, requires little oversight.
4	1. Averages [X] patient encounters per hour. 2. Makes decisions about diagnosis and treatment almost completely autonomously. 3. Performs procedures almost completely autonomously.
5	1. Maintains panel of at least [X] patients. 2. Diagnoses and manages clinically complex patients with little assistance. 3. Has attained additional certification for performing [service/procedure]. 4. Accepts on-call responsibilities in rotation.
6	1. Maintains panel of at least [X] patients. 2. Diagnoses and manages clinically complex patients autonomously. 3. Participates in ER coverage rotation.
7	1. Maintains panel of at least [X] patients. 2. Diagnoses and manages clinically complex patients autonomously. 3. Responsible for oversight of other midlevel providers.

PROFESSIONAL SKILLS

Skill Detail	Description
1	1. Has not developed full competency on systems (EHR, PACS, etc.). 2. Still regularly asks OS or others how things work before referencing onboarding documents, equipment manuals etc. 3. Refers patients prematurely. 4. Is still developing rapport with patients.
2	1. Has developed working proficiency with practice systems. 2. Always willing to help in areas outside of responsibility when needed. 3. Asks for feedback in manner that makes it easy to give ("How could I have done that better?"). 4. Owns responsibility for making mistakes and says he/she is sorry ("I screwed that one up and I'm really sorry about it. I think I could have avoided it or done better next time by…"). 5. Seeks out opportunities for clinical learning. 6. Doesn't view current amount of knowledge as "enough" — seeks to acquire new skills.
3	1. Has demonstrated the ability to identify what is wrong with a "quietly unhappy" patient. 2. Uses practice systems proficiently. 3. Regularly looks for ways to increase efficiency with patient flow, systems, and processes. 4. Regularly receives verbal and written praise from patients. 5. Refers patients appropriately 6. Demonstrates awareness of quality of care metrics and regularly meets them. 7. Speaks with poise and confidence to patients, coworkers, and referring providers.
4	1. Shares ideas about how [Organization] could improve in an actionable manner. 2. Has learned enough about how systems and processes work that can problem solve when issues arise. 3. Almost always meets CMS quality of care metrics. 4. Maintains a good working relationship with coworkers and staff. 5. Committed to a self-study program, reading books/journals and skill development.
5	1. Known as a leader informally among coworkers and staff. 2. Participates in activities to increase awareness of [Organization] such as marketing events or speaking opportunities. 3. Cited as a valuable resource for colleagues. 4. Known for anticipating and solving problems before they develop. 5. Has earned a [professional title, certification etc.] designation.
6	1. Has become known in community for "wow" service levels, leading to regular positive feedback from patients. 2. Holds a formal leadership role within the practice. 3. Mentors others, in and out of similar roles. Cited as valuable resource by people throughout [Organization].

CHAPTER 7

Recruiting and Retaining Midlevel Providers

Cut costs and run a healthy business

Responsible for the operation of 14 primary care sites, the chief medical officer of a community health system in Los Angeles had extensive experience working with advanced practice providers. Given the number of clinic locations within the health system, I anticipated the company could benefit from a residency-like program for nurse practitioners interested in working with underserved populations.

I was surprised when the physician CMO told me that, unlike other area community health facilities, her health system did not have problems with staffing. In fact, they maintained very low turnover rates among midlevel providers. Curious about how the practice accomplished such stability, I asked for her secret. The CMO attributed the company's impressive retention statistics primarily to a well-developed onboarding program and process.

The health system recognized that the way midlevel providers began their employment dictated the tone of the relationship long term. Not only did the company emphasize onboarding, it also committed to finding the right person for the job rather than finding the person with the right type of practice experience. As a result, new midlevel hires primarily were motivated, high-achieving new graduate nurse practitioners.

Upon starting at the practice, the newly hired NP began a standardized, systematized onboarding process. After an initial training and brief shadowing period, the nurse practitioner's schedule was set at 8 patients per day. Not only was patient volume kept low for the new NP, the new provider was also supported by a physician mentor. The nurse practitioner gradually increased patient volume, from 8 to 12 patients per day, incrementally adding to the schedule with the ultimate goal of seeing 17 patients per day by the end of the six-month onboarding period.

The physician mentor assisted with questions that presented throughout the workday, helping the NP grow in clinical competence and confidence. Midlevel providers who went through this process didn't leave the practice. Furthermore, the CMO stated that the onboarding system provided quality control. Structured oversight allowed physicians to give clinical input, training the NP to work at the standard required in the practice and in line with the company's culture.

This particular community health system stands out as one with an exceptional process for integrating midlevel providers into its practices, yet many practices fail to maintain quality employment relationships with midlevel providers. Implementing systems and processes for successfully recruiting, onboarding, and maintaining midlevel providers requires foresight and effort. In the end, however, time spent on implementing these processes is well worth the effort. It results in less turnover and a more stable and therefore profitable practice.

THE SIGNIFICANCE OF TURNOVER

A provider vacancy is a big deal for your practice. Not only does it leave your patients in a lurch, affecting the customer service and care you're able to provide, it is also quite costly. Ultimately, it can take several months to fill a vacant midlevel provider position, which means significant missed revenue for your practice. Additionally, when you do hire a new provider, you must invest the time to train that individual and to transition your patients and staff as well.

The True Cost of Turnover

Although hiring midlevel providers, particularly those with less experience, may not seem to be worth the time and energy required to train them, filling a position quickly and retaining that provider proves beneficial.

A vacant NP position *conservatively* costs your clinic $1,500/day or more in missed revenue potential. Consider a scenario where a nurse practitioner works eight hours/day treating three patients per hour. If these patient visits are each assigned a 99213, basic office visit CPT code, and the visit is billed to Medicare, the NP stands to generate about $1,490 in revenue for the clinic each day. This doesn't even begin to take into account revenue for ancillary services or visits billed with more complex CPT codes. Missed revenue due to a hiring delay is even higher.

The longer the position remains open, the more money your practice stands to lose. For businesses that fail to fill job openings within the first month, there is a 57% chance that the position will remain open for three months or more.[1] Assuming the scenario above, a nurse practitioner position left open for three months results in $89,352 or more in missed revenue.

The Center for American Progress estimates that turnover costs businesses just over 20% of a position's annual salary.[2] The organization notes that the cost of turnover for positions requiring a specific skill set, such as those of medical providers, is much higher.

The *New England Journal of Medicine* estimates the cost of physician turnover at over $1 million when taking missed revenue into account.[3] While the hiring costs and revenue generated by midlevel providers are lower than those for physicians, employers can still expect midlevel turnover to have financial implications, possibly well into the six-figure range. Costs associated with midlevel provider turnover may include sign-on bonuses, relocation expenses, recruiting fees, administrative time and interview costs, as well as the time of staff members.

While finances are an obvious consideration in evaluating the cost of a vacant midlevel provider position, it's important to consider other effects as well. Each time an employee leaves, relationships with patients and coworkers are severed. This affects customer service and workplace culture. The effect may manifest itself as decreased morale among staff, now overworked to compensate for the additional responsibilities left by the vacancy.

Or, turnover may mean losing patients to a competing practice. In a healthcare environment where patient satisfaction is increasingly tied to reimbursement, maintaining stable patient-provider relationships becomes even more valuable.

Few practices recognize the true financial and cultural impact of turnover among nurse practitioners and physician assistants. Even fewer recognize the difference that setting appropriate expectations and investing time in training and supporting midlevel providers can make.

THE TURNOVER SOLUTION

In the *American Journal of Medical Quality's Review of Physician Turnover: Rates, Causes and Consequences*, the authors report that 54% of physicians leave their practice within five years. The most commonly cited reason for departure (30% of cases) is "broken promises" regarding patient volume and administrative support.[4] In a related survey, 74% of employers indicate that they believe providing mentorship to physicians would reduce turnover. Despite this recognition, only 56% of respondents assign a mentor to new physicians.[5] While these studies surveyed physicians, we can expect trends surrounding the relationship between support, mentorship and turnover among midlevel providers to look similar.

Based on the findings of these surveys, it seems that practices know what needs to be done, but don't follow through. Employers recognize that mentorship reduces turnover, saving tens or even hundreds of thousands of dollars for each prevented loss, however they don't implement systems to provide such support.

As an employer, you can't expect to maintain the status quo and get different results. Adequate support and training are key components to preventing the hassle and financial burden of turnover among advanced practice providers. Investing time and resources on the front end of the employment relationship is necessary to prevent future losses.

Encouraging longevity with your practice starts with transparency about job expectations and compensation. It also means following a few core principles for supporting and maintaining relationships with midlevel providers.

Principle 1: Communication

Communication is at the core of any relationship. Poor communication commonly is cited as a top reason couples split up. While you aren't looking for a soulmate in your next hire, you will be spending a significant amount of time with that individual and place a piece of the responsibility for your company's success on his or her shoulders. So, it makes sense that you should take the time to lay out expectations for the provider's role up front. Not only does this mitigate conflict and employment dissatisfaction, it also sets the tone for open and honest communication in the future.

As you convey roles and responsibilities of the midlevel provider during the interview process, use your compensation levels document as a guide and share it with your prospect. This way you won't neglect to include important details. Setting 30, 60, and 90-day goals for your new hire is another way to ensure communication about expectations. As part of your onboarding process, set expectations for what a new provider should accomplish during each of these timeframes. Don't neglect to set a time for follow-up and feedback on these metrics.

Additionally, turn the tables and think about the job from the prospective provider's perspective. What do you wish you had known before accepting the position with your practice? What challenges do you anticipate the provider will face in the initial months of employment? Are there any upcoming changes within the company that will affect the provider's job? Address these types of issues in the interview process. Most people welcome a challenge or two, provided the circumstance was expected and communicated.

I recently talked with a nurse practitioner, Karen, who was struggling in her practice. As a recent graduate, Karen sought a position supportive of her inexperience. The physician who hired her paired her with an experienced NP who was willing to provide training in the clinical setting.

Another term of Karen's employment was the expectation of a graduated patient volume. She would see significantly fewer patients than other providers in the practice, increasing her numbers slowly as she became more knowledgeable. Fairly, her salary would be at the lower end of the spectrum, increasing as she gained proficiency. The employment relationship seemed poised for success as the employer and new hire had clearly laid out expectations.

Things went smoothly as Karen came on board. The clinical support system in place and patient volume expectations were challenging but manageable. From the practice's perspective, Karen's employment was still profitable and showed promise of trending upward in the coming months.

After a few weeks, however, she began to encounter resistance. Staff members, including nurses, medical assistants, and the scheduling manager, had not been made aware of the expectations for the new provider. Comments about how Karen wasn't seeing many patients or pulling her own weight were degrading. The scheduling manager constantly pushed her to see more patients even though she was already finishing up work after hours.

The expectations for her as a new NP set in place by administrators were not communicated to support staff and therefore often breeched when they inconvenienced these staff members.

Roles, expectations, and responsibilities that affect others must be clearly communicated to these staff members. If you as an employer present a certain expectation as far as patient volume, but neglect to share this with the individual in charge of scheduling, for example, the term you agreed upon is likely to fail.

If you commit to being a supportive workplace for midlevel providers with less experience, the expectation that experienced providers must assist NPs and PAs with a positive attitude must also be clear. Providers and staff don't work in isolation. Clear communication about each individual's role is essential to following through on these expectations. Fewer surprises means an all-around better employment experience for everyone on your team.

Principle 2: Training and Mentoring

Experienced or otherwise, nurse practitioners and physician assistants in your practice must have an adequate support system in place. This support system starts the first day on the job. Consider the best way for the provider to learn the ropes in your practice. The temptation with more experienced providers will be to assume that since the clinical role is similar to the provider's previous experience, little onboarding is necessary. While primary care looks similar across the profession, for example, the way it is provided varies.

What will the new provider need to know as far as day-to-day practice operations, such as the EMR system or patient resources? Are there any communication norms the provider should be aware of when it comes to interacting with staff and patients? What resources are available for patients who cannot afford traditional healthcare services?

Often, I talk with nurse practitioners and physician assistants who step into a new job and find the process overwhelming. Some of this is expected with a change in employment, but, the process could be made simpler and less chaotic with foresight and planning.

Take the time to introduce the new hire to staff members. Make sure they know where to find things and how to access resources. Literally show them the bathroom. These things seem intuitive, but far too many practices skip them. Create a written process for onboarding so that none of these steps is missed.

Less-experienced midlevel providers will also need additional support in the clinical aspect of their role. Consider a brief job-shadowing period so the new NP or PA can become familiar with how other providers in your facility practice. Make sure that more experienced providers are aware of the expectation for training and supporting the new NP or PA in the clinical setting and that they are willing to facilitate this continued learning process.

Consider implementing a formal structure for how clinical support of midlevel providers will occur in your practice. In the emergency department where I work, for example, physicians take shifts being the go-to for midlevels. Every four hours, the supporting MD role is transferred to another physician. The schedule is clearly outlined and posted in the provider work area to eliminate any confusion. Other practices take the approach of pairing each midlevel provider with a physician assigned as a mentor for that provider. This physician serves as a support system, making himself or herself available to the midlevel provider.

Decide what support should look like in your practice, then establish a system for implementing this structure.

Principle 3: Work-Life Balance

Burnout has become a buzzword in medicine. But, as one who was once a sleep-deprived, over-committed full-time nurse practitioner who sought career balance by starting my own business, I understand the reality of the phenomenon. We're working ourselves until we hate our jobs. Subject to pressures from the government and administrators, we're becoming increasingly dissatisfied with our careers as healthcare providers. Surveys consistently show, for example, that more than 40% of doctors would not choose medicine if they had to do it all over again.

Preventing employee burnout can be difficult. Interacting with patients in short periods of time over the course of a full work week is demanding, but, it's how you generate revenue. Complying with the ever-increasing list of patient care guidelines produced by government agencies is challenging, but, it's tied to compensation. And, yes, it's nearly impossible to adopt flexible schedules and lenient time-off policies that are popular with many progressive employers; patient care for the most part demands in-person interaction.

So, as an employer, how do you give providers the work-life balance they're looking for?

Keeping midlevel providers happy in their roles begins with shielding them from the confusion and mismanagement the government has forced onto healthcare. Avoid compensating providers based on productivity; this eliminates the exhausting game of keeping score and the anxiety of a variable paycheck. Rather, make compensation and corresponding expectations clear. Set the bar for performance high and keep it consistent. Predictability in employment is comforting.

Protect providers from the stress associated with government whims so they can focus on meeting the metrics you as an employer deem most important to success.

Another mistake employers commonly make is treating nurse practitioners and physician assistants like residents. While midlevel providers may not be physicians, they are not there to be dumped on, made to feel inferior, or to be dealt only undesirable work hours—unless that is the up-front expectation of employment.

Many midlevel providers considered careers as physicians, ultimately choosing to avoid the lifestyle that comes with the demands of residency and ultimate patient care responsibility. Their compensation reflects this different scope of responsibility.

The medical model of training certainly has its benefits. In some ways, you may find that working with a less-experienced midlevel provider feels similar to working with a resident. Be respectful, however, of the expectations set at the beginning of employment so that the NP doesn't burnout.

Finally, check in with nurse practitioners and physician assistants as part of regular, formal feedback sessions. This allows you to assess for signs of stress and job dissatisfaction. It also provides a forum for addressing concerns or performance issues.

A few years ago, the emergency department where I work was going through some staffing transitions; in addition, a nurse practitioner was away on medical leave. This left significant gaps in the provider schedule. I had always tried to help during times of need, so the medical director asked if I could take on a few extra shifts. I did. The slim staffing situation in the ED dragged on, and I continued to work overtime for two more months. While the substantial paycheck was appreciated, constant transitions from night shift to day shift with little time in between was wearing on me in a big way.

One day, the medical director saw me in the hallway and asked how I was doing. In a foggy, sleep-deprived state, I began to cry. And I'm not a crier. We stepped into his office to discuss the issue and I said that I wanted to help out but was struggling to keep up with the demands of working extra hours.

To solve the problem, the medical director temporarily allowed physicians to cover some of the open midlevel shifts, alleviating the NPs and PAs on staff of what had become a growing burden. The quick response to my feedback (and uncharacteristic breakdown) swiftly reversed the growing grumblings among the midlevel provider team, restoring job satisfaction. Had the medical director not been receptive to my feedback, employees would have quit.

Check in regularly with each individual on your provider team. It's more effective if these sessions are formally scheduled in advance. Ask midlevel providers to submit an agenda of what they think are the most important things to discuss in the meeting. Add your own items to the agenda as well, and share the complete itemized list before you meet. This way, everyone can prepare their thoughts about each item before you meet.

Regularly scheduled feedback allows you to detect problems early and clues you in as to small changes you might make to facilitate work-life balance for your employees. On the flip side, it also gives you the opportunity to share with providers how they measure up on performance metrics and offer steps for improvement.

Principle 4: Workplace Culture

Preventing turnover and burnout among midlevel providers begins with setting a positive tone for your practice. This tone dictates how members of the team interact with one another and with their patients. So-called workplace culture is the authentic "feel" of your practice and can positively or negatively impact your company's productivity. It guides decision making and influences the level of pride employees take in their work.

A positive culture inspires and gives meaning to day-to-day activities. Culture and norms develop organically whether you are aware of them or not. Employers must intentionally set the pulse of the company in a positive direction and maintain this feel and vision in face of changes and challenges.

Create a Positive Culture

How do you intentionally create a positive culture for your practice?

First, evaluate your current practice culture. If you could describe your practice with five adjectives, what would they be? Would these be the same words your employees use to describe your company?

Second, determine your company's values. Why does your practice exist? What do you do well that similar practices do not? What sets you apart from other healthcare facilities? What do you wish set you apart? As you go through this exercise, think about the way you would like to describe your practice and how it sets itself apart from the thousands of other businesses in your specialty. These descriptors allow you to identify your company's values and determine what your practice culture will look like.

Once you have outlined your ideal practice culture, you can begin to influence the behaviors of providers and staff to help build this culture.

Share Your Vision

To inspire other physicians, midlevel providers, and staff, you must share the company's vision with everyone. Paint a picture of why your practice exists and what sets it apart from others. Describe how the care you provide impacts individual patients and your community. Discuss the vision for the company and any plans for growth or other goals for the business.

People want to contribute to something larger than themselves. Letting providers and other staff in on the company outlook shows them how to contribute to accomplish this greater goal and gives purpose to everyday activities.

Focus on Organizational Design

Culture starts with the systems, processes, and organizational hierarchy you put into place as an employer. These structures guide day-to-day operations, dictating how employees interact as well as how efficiently and smoothly they can do their jobs. An organization focused on hierarchy, for example, will be more formal. One with a more collaborative structure encourages teamwork. A practice without norms in place for how patients are assigned to providers may experience dissension or foster competition among providers.

In addition to creating a reporting structure, you also must be intentional about establishing systems around which daily activities are carried out. Practices with a structure for how patients are assigned and distributed among providers, for example, will be a collaborative workplace with a greater spirit of cooperation.

Hire with Purpose

Healthcare practices must structure their hiring processes. This ensures that not only NPs and PAs, but also other providers and staff are a good cultural fit for the workplace.

Some healthcare groups are laid back, others highly driven. Some practices are focused on revenue, others on relationships with patients and serving the community.

Intelligence, talent, and experience don't necessarily mean an NP or PA is a good fit for your team. Consider how an individual will integrate into your workplace culture as you bring new employees on board.

Maintain Open Communication

Regular feedback helps maintain an open line of communication with midlevel providers. The same is true among other members of your team. Consider starting each week with a 10-minute Monday morning meet-up for all staff members to get everyone on the same page about what needs to be accomplished or any upcoming changes for the week. You might even consider starting each day with a 10-minute check in. Beginning the day as a group sets the tone for teamwork, not to mention eliminates tardy arrivals.

Regular communication keeps employees engaged in the success of the practice. It reinforces the vision you have laid out for your future as a company. It keeps employees accountable and encourages ownership of responsibilities. Reporting progress on meeting a metric in front of one's boss, for example, applies less pressure than reporting progress in front of peers and the practice as a whole.

Be Professionally Positive

Constructive criticism and negative feedback are certainly warranted at times. Too often, we save communication only for these moments. Don't neglect to celebrate the accomplishments of midlevel providers in your practice. This encourages achievement and helps those who are high performers maintain motivation. When problems do arise, refrain from addressing the problem in unprofessional or punitive ways. Gossip and negative side comments or conversations are counterproductive to creating a culture that fosters positive relationships.

Set Transparent Expectations

Maintaining transparency around expectations for midlevel providers and others on your team is a core component of company culture. Without this foundation, providers are kept guessing as to what is expected of them. This opens the door to dissatisfaction and disappointment, a slippery slope that may destroy the work you have put into building your practice's culture.

IN SUMMARY

There is an old business adage that goes something like this:

CFO asks CEO: What happens if we spend time and money training our people and they leave?

CEO: What happens if we don't and they stay?

Developing and implementing systems and processes around how you recruit, hire, and train midlevel providers sound like a lot of work. And it is, at first. Once you get these systems in place, however, they lead to quality employment relationships and prevent turnover in your practice, an issue far more time consuming and detrimental to your business.

Applying these four principles to recruiting and maintaining relationships with mid-level providers sounds intuitive, yet, most practices fail to implement such structures. Set yourself and your practice apart by taking the time and effort required to create a standout culture and watch as the dynamics and productivity of your company begin to change.

REFERENCES

1. Time to Fill Jobs in the US: The 30 Day Tipping Point. Indeed. January 2015. Retrieved September 3, 2016, from http://press.indeed.com/wp-content/uploads/2015/01/Time-to-fill-jobs-in-the-US.pdf.
2. Westgate A. The high cost of medical practice staff turnover. *Physicians Practice*. June 21, 2013. Retrieved September 12, 2016, from www.physicianspractice.com/blog/high-cost-medical-practice-staff-turnover.
3. Schute L. Understanding the real costs of recruiting. *Recruiting Physicians Today 2012; 20*(3):1 Retrieved from www.nejmcareercenter.org/minisites/rpt/understanding-the-real-costs-of-recruiting/.
4. Misra-Hebert AD., Kay R., & Stoller J. K. A review of physician turnover: rates, causes, and consequences. *Am J Med Qual 2004; 19*(2):56-66.
5. Fierce Healthcare. How much is physician turnover really costing you? Fierce Healthcare. August 4, 2011. Retrieved October 14, 2016, from www.fiercehealthcare.com/healthcare/how-much-physician-turnover-really-costing-you.

CHAPTER 8

Final Considerations for Using Advanced Practice Providers

Putting the finishing touches on your playbook

Many facilities hesitate to integrate nurse practitioners and physician assistants into their practices for a variety of reasons. Common hesitations center around the following topics:

1. Efficacy: "How much will physician productivity suffer?"
2. Integration: "I've tried and it doesn't work."
3. Malpractice: "How will hiring a midlevel provider affect my liability?"

Integrating nurse practitioners and physician assistants into a practice isn't for everyone. However, for those concerned about these aspects of employing advanced practice providers, data and case studies provide insight into these concerns. In addition, practices can use several strategies to mitigate these risks and challenges.

EFFICACY: PHYSICIAN PRODUCTIVITY AND MIDLEVEL PROVIDERS

Two financial metrics are important to consider when it comes to employing midlevel providers in your practice: the direct and indirect financial impacts.

To quantify the direct cost or value of employing midlevel providers, simply calculate anticipated or actual revenue the provider brings to the practice compared with the cost of employing that provider.

With regard to the direct financial implications of bringing on a midlevel provider, the numbers are favorable. For example, results of a 2011 survey by the American Academy of Orthopedic Surgeons indicate that nurse practitioners and physician assistants are compensated on average between $85,000 and $95,000 annually. At the same time, collections for these providers range between $147,000 and $175,000. A 2014 Medical Group Management Association report had similar findings, showing that practices utilizing advanced practice providers perform better financially and generate higher revenues.[1] Overall, employing NPs and PAs is a revenue-generating decision.

The indirect financial impacts of employing midlevel providers are more difficult to quantify. Many practices worry that one detriment of using NPs and PAs will be reduced physician productivity. Employing advanced practice providers effectively requires modified systems, processes, and a management structure. Physicians worry that spending time on administrative tasks and providing clinical support to advanced practice providers will affect their ability to see patients. In turn, seeing fewer patients equates to lower clinical productivity and less time for revenue-generating activities.

When we look at how midlevel providers affect physician productivity, however, it's essential to look at the practice as a whole. Supervising a nurse practitioner may take time away from individual physicians' ability to see patients. Having another provider on board, however, positively impacts productivity and revenue overall.

A group of physicians practicing at the Mayo Clinic decided to explore the financial impact of using "physician extenders"— nurse practitioners and physician assistants—in their practices.[3] Recognizing that the number of hours spent by physicians on patient care is decreasing while practice overhead is increasing, the group tested a model in which physician extenders helped complete non-billable work on behalf of physicians.[2]

Prior to the study, each of the group's eight physicians spent a total of 84 minutes per physician per day performing indirect patient care. The results of the study were staggering. Employing a physician extender for just four hours a day, five days a week, reduced physician indirect patient care by one hour per physician per day. Doctors went from spending nearly an hour and a half on non-billable activities to less than 30 minutes per day.

Authors of the study note that expanding the physician extenders' hours would have had an even greater impact on these results. Physicians spending less time on indirect patient care were able to allot more time to billable patient care, research, and education.

Time spent after regular work hours also decreased for those using a physician extender, compared with the control group in the study. Most surprising of all, RVU-based patient care productivity (RVU/out-patient physician/day) increased 41% for physicians using the physician extender compared with just 18% for the control group over the course of the study.

In *Today's Hospitalist*, Dr. David Friar, CEO of Hospitalists of Northwest Michigan, a 50-provider group, echoes these sentiments about employing midlevel providers. "Many groups approach adding midlevels as a way to boost revenue and that's a big mistake; the involvement of NPs improves the entire group's function, so it's not about billing," he says.

NPs and PAs in the group do have patient care responsibilities. However, they also are expected to chip in when it comes to non-billable activities, including acting as enforcers of core-compliance measures and other administrative responsibilities. "It makes much more sense to be using midlevels who earn $64 an hour as hospitalist representatives throughout the hospital, than having a physician earning $250 an hour doing big-time committee work. Who's the cheapest guy to send?" he reasons.[23]

Healthcare providers spend excessive amounts of time on job responsibilities for which they cannot bill. Implementing a model whereby nurse practitioners and physician assistants are able to take on some of these responsibilities frees up time for physicians billing at higher rates to focus on revenue-generating activities. Not to mention, non-billable types of tasks are often those that physicians enjoy the least.

While on-the-job training and mentoring midlevel providers certainly takes a bite out of a physician's schedule, ultimately the time freed up by the NP or PA helping out in other capacities outweighs this time investment.

INTEGRATION: DEVELOPING A PLAYBOOK

My three-year-old nephew was enrolled in a soccer program. On Saturday mornings during soccer season, my brother-in-law often texted us video clips of the games—typically a hoard of preschoolers chasing the ball in a tight pack, tripping over one another's feet. Passing the ball was a distant thought as the one-track strategy was to get the ball, keep it, and take it to the net.

Young children don't often understand the concept that working as a team with a strategy is more effective and efficient than going at it alone. The playbooks of college teams, in contrast, define the role and responsibilities of each player, allowing for significantly greater overall achievement on the field.

Many of our healthcare facilities and provider groups operate in a manner similar to that of young children's sports teams. Am I saying that NPs and PAs are like three-year-olds? Of course not. However, too often we expect providers to perform but neglect to give them a framework for success. We hire providers without a plan to bring them on board and integrate them into our practices. It's not surprising, then, that many practices fail to successfully implement nurse practitioners and physician assistants into their business models.

One objection I commonly hear from physicians when it comes to hiring NPs and PAs is "We've tried and it doesn't work" or "So-and-so tried and it didn't work." My follow up to this objection is "Show me your playbook."

If you hire advanced practice providers without doing your homework, you can expect failure. If you haven't done due diligence when it comes to plotting the financial trajectory of your practice or implementing a process by which you will onboard and measure the performance of providers, you might as well be trying to win a high caliber sports contest without a playbook.

How will your team know where the practice's priorities lie? Without a clear message about expectations for employment, each provider will pursue what he or she deems to be most important. These efforts may contribute to or be misaligned with the mission and goals of your practice. It's up to you to put your team members on the right track.

Creating your Playbook

In essence, this book serves as a guide to getting started with your playbook. The act of creating a compensation levels document delineates the role and responsibilities of advanced practice providers on your team, significantly impacting the chance of success with advanced practice providers. Furthermore, standardized hiring practices optimize the caliber of NPs and PAs in your practice. Businesses are built on people, and attracting the right players to your practice is a critical component of success.

There are a few additional challenges practices face when integrating NPs and PAs into their business models that should be addressed in your playbook. These include:

1. Restrictive payment policies
2. Scope of practice laws
3. Scheduling
4. Documentation/coding
5. Clinical knowledge

It's essential to consider these factors as you develop a plan for integrating NPs and PAs into your practice.

Restrictive payment policies. Before you hop on board the midlevel provider band-wagon, make sure you'll be reimbursed for it. Payers are different in every state and influence the value a nurse practitioner or physician assistant adds to your practice. New Jersey's Medicaid program, for example, reimburses advanced practice providers at 95% of non-specialist physician fees. In contrast, Indiana's Medicaid program reimburses advanced practice providers at just 75% of physician rates.[4] Build your financial model accurately by understanding the policies of payers in your area.

Cheryl Toth, senior practice management professional, also recommends survey-ing private payers when it comes to billing guidelines. "Despite the fact that Medicare has clear and specific billing rules, many private payers don't" she says. Toth advises contacting your top 10 private payers and asking about billing, reimbursement rates, and payment guidelines for advanced practice providers. "Organize the information into a written document so the billing office is clear about the rules and the practice has 'institutional memory' beyond just the person who made the calls," she advises.[5]

You also will want to familiarize yourself with billing loopholes, such as Medicare's incident-to stipulation. This way of billing for out-patient healthcare services allows the midlevel provider to bill under the physician's provider number and to be reimbursed at 100% of the physician rate for the encounter. Incident-to billing gets complicated in that to apply, the physician must be in the office and the patient must be a follow-up visit for an established problem. Decide if the complexity of navigating such caveats and maximizing reimbursement is worth it for your facility. Identify additional reimburse-ment policies that can work to your advantage given your patient population.

Scope of practice laws. Investigate your state's scope of practice laws—they will affect the way you're allowed to utilize nurse practitioners and physician assistants. Florida nurse practitioners, for example, only gained the right to prescribe controlled substances on January 1, 2017. Historically, this restriction greatly limited the utility of NPs in the state. In Missouri, nurse practitioners are required to practice within a 30-mile radius of a collaborating physician, a limitation for some practices. In California, physicians are limited as to the number of NPs and PAs they may oversee at any given time.

How will scope of practice laws affect your ability to integrate advanced practice providers into your practice? Before moving forward with hiring midlevel providers, it's important to ask:

1. Will hiring a nurse practitioner, physician assistant, or either be more beneficial given scope of practice guidelines?
2. How will my staffing model need to look based on any limitations placed on NPs or PAs by state law?

Considering state law optimizes the benefit that hiring a midlevel provider will have for your practice and ensures there aren't any unforeseen hurdles once the decision has been made.

Scheduling. Based on my experience partnering with a number of facilities as they integrate nurse practitioners and physician assistants into their practices, scheduling seems to be a repeat offender when it comes to implementation. Staff may be unfamiliar with the advanced practice provider role or unclear as to what types of patients the nurse practitioner or physician assistant is to treat.

Recently, a nurse practitioner contacted me to talk about scheduling at the practice where she worked. As part of her agreement with the practice, she was to see a specified low volume of patients per day in her initial months of employment while she developed her clinical skill set. She was frustrated because individuals in charge of scheduling repeatedly overrode her scheduling parameters to add additional patients to her load. The chief medical officer who hired her and determined the terms of her employment had failed to communicate these to support staff.

Whenever you bring on a new nurse practitioner or physician assistant, familiarize those responsible for scheduling with the game plan. This is especially important if the advanced practice providers will be assigned patients in a different manner than physicians. Develop a fool-proof system for assigning patients in your practice.

Documentation and coding. Right or wrong, in most cases as a healthcare provider, you're paid according to your documentation. Incomplete or inadequate documentation will cost you. We've all heard the phrase "if it wasn't documented, it wasn't done." Nurse practitioners and physician assistants receive notoriously little guidance when it comes to billing and coding in their education programs. Give these providers guidance on documentation to maximize reimbursement. Review charts regularly, looking for areas where the NP or PA can improve. Teach midlevel providers how to get paid for the work that they do.

Clinical knowledge. As discussed throughout this book, it's likely that the midlevel provider you bring into your practice will need some clinical training. New graduates will require significantly more assistance than those with experience. Experienced NPs and PAs may require specialized procedural knowledge or may need to build upon foundational clinical skills.

Maintain clear expectations regarding the individuals responsible for providing clinical support to midlevel providers in your practice. If certain skills are essential to the function of NPs and PAs in your facility, provide training for these skills as part of your structured onboarding process. Neglecting to devote time and resources to advancing midlevel provider's clinical skills means you won't utilize these providers to their maximum potential.

MIDLEVEL PROVIDERS AND MALPRACTICE

Working with nurse practitioners and physician assistants naturally raises concerns about liability. Will you be held liable for the actions of midlevel providers in your practice? If your employment arrangement, facility, or state laws mandate physician supervision of advanced practice providers, then as a physician, you are ultimately responsible for the care they provide, even if you are not directly involved in treating the patient. If the NP or PA working under you is sued, you will be as well.

Litigation against nurse practitioners and physician assistants is on the rise with the growing numbers of NPs and PAs entering the profession. However, analysis of the trend shows that the rate of malpractice payments is steady and consistent with the growth in the number of providers.

Perhaps the most insightful information we have on the impact of NPs and PAs on medical malpractice liability comes from a 2009 *Journal of Medical Licensure and Discipline* study. In the study, authors compiled 17 years' worth of data from the United States National Provider Databank (NPDB) looking at malpractice incidence, payment amount, and other measures of liability among physicians and advanced practice providers. Throughout the 17 years of study data, there was an average of one malpractice payment report for every 2.7 active physicians, one for every 32.5 active PAs, and just one for every 65.8 active NPs. In percentage terms, 37% of physicians, 3.1% of PAs, and 1.5% of NPs would have made a malpractice payment during that 17-year period.

Based on this data, authors of the study conclude that "There were no observations or trends to suggest that PAs and NPs increase liability. If anything, they may decrease the rate of reporting malpractice and adverse events."[6]

Why do nurse practitioners and physician assistants enjoy significantly decreased liability compared to physicians? Advanced practice providers are less likely to be seen as "deep pockets" and in turn are less likely to be targeted with a malpractice suit. Authors in the 2009 study also note that nurse practitioners tend to spend more time with their patients than physicians, building a higher degree of rapport and allowing for improved patient-provider communication.

Finally, the role of advanced practice providers is continuing to develop. Given that midlevel providers' scope of practice is somewhat limited, this reduces exposure to liability. As the level of autonomy with which NPs and PAs are allowed to practice increases, the rate of medical malpractice payouts will as well.

Given the inherent liability that accompanies working alongside nurse practitioners and physician assistants, it is essential that physicians, NPs, and PAs practice with an awareness of these risks and take steps to mitigate them.

In *Medical Practice Management*, attorney Barbara Paterick states that negligence is the most common form of malpractice action taken against healthcare providers.[7] As it relates to claims against physicians for negligence on part of the midlevel provider, these are typically based on errors related to:

1. Lack of adequate supervision by the physician;
2. Tardy or absent referral of subspecialty care;
3. Incorrect diagnosis or failure to identify the correct diagnosis;
4. Physical exam or evaluation that is cursory or not performed;
5. Misrepresentation of the credentials of the provider; and
6. Lack of due diligence in hiring the provider.

By addressing each of these items, practices can implement norms to decrease the risk of liability in their practices.

Lack of Adequate Supervision

When it comes to supervision, two primary conditions must be met:

1. The activity is within the scope of practice of the individual performing the task; and
2. The individual performing the task is qualified and properly trained.

First and foremost, practices must examine supervision relating to state laws. Do the laws in your state specify the way supervision must occur? In Tennessee, where I practice, for example, a collaborating physician must review 20% of the nurse practitioner's charts. In Missouri, nurse practitioners must practice within a 30 to 50-mile radius of the supervising physician, depending on the practice setting. Yet other states may limit the number of advanced practice providers a physician may supervise at any given time. Compliance with state laws decreases liability risk.

Addressing proper training and qualifications of advanced practice providers is where the principles outlined in this book come into play. With well-documented systems and processes for hiring and onboarding nurse practitioner and physician assistants, you can rest assured that the midlevel providers in your practice meet practice standards. Should a provider's actions be called into question, you may also reference these onboarding standards as evidence of qualifications.

Misrepresentation of Provider Credentials

Misrepresentation occurs when the patient is not informed that the advanced practice provider is not a physician. The increasing popularity of the Doctor of Nursing Practice (DNP) degree for nurse practitioners increases the likelihood of misrepresentation. NPs with doctoral level degrees may introduce themselves as "Dr. ___", but must also include their designation as a nurse practitioner in their introduction. Individuals responsible for scheduling appointments must inform patients that they will be seeing an advanced practice provider to eliminate any confusion about the provider's credentials. Setting a norm for your practice that providers introduce themselves to each patient by name and title mitigates misrepresentation risk.

Hiring Due Diligence

Physicians and healthcare employers must use due diligence in hiring decisions, particularly when it comes to midlevel providers. This includes verifying education, experience, and licensure. Querying the National Provider Databank will also alert you to any disciplinary action taken against the provider that he or she has failed to disclose.

IN SUMMARY

These common concerns surrounding the integration of advanced practice providers in your practice are valid. There is risk inherent to modifying your practice model and bringing additional providers on board. Norms for the role of NPs and PAs in your practice and a clear structure for oversight, however, increase your chance of success while reducing liability risk.

REFERENCES

1. McKesson Business Performance Services. Non-physician providers can ease clinical burden, boost practice revenue. McKesson. Retrieved January 19, 2017, from http://www.mckesson.com/bps/blog/non-physician-providers-can-ease-clinical-burden-boost-practice-revenue/
2. Rodysill KJ. Increasing physician productivity using a physician extender: A study in an outpatient group practice at the Mayo Clinic. *J Med Pract Manage* 2003; Sep-Oct 19(2):110-14.
3. Darves B. Success with midlevels: How does your group stack up? *Today's Hospitalist*. July 2010. Retrieved February 2, 2017, from www.todayshospitalist.com/success-with-midlevels-how-does-your-group-stack-up/.
4. Medicaid Benefits: Nurse Practitioner Services. *The Henry J. Kaiser Family Foundation*. 2012. Retrieved February 5, 2017, from http://kff.org/medicaid/state-indicator/nurse-practitioner-services/?currentTimeframe=0.
5. Toth, C. Seven surefire ways to start a nonphysician practitioner off right. *J Med Pract Manage*. 2014 Jan-Feb;29(4): 214-15.
6. Hooker RS, Nicholson J, & Le T. (2009). Does the employment of physician assistants and nurse practitioners increase liability? *Journal of Medical Licensure and Discipline*. 2009;95(2):6-16.
7. Paterick, BB, Waterhouse BE, Paterick, TE, & Sanbar, SS. Liability of physicians supervising nonphysician clinicians. *J Med Pract Manage*. 2014 Mar-Apr;29(5):309-13.

CHAPTER 9

A Flawed System—How Did We Get Here?

A brief timeline of the U.S. healthcare system and its impact on medical providers

Most of our medical practices are set up in a way more conducive to patient dissatisfaction than to customer service, more to burnout than productivity. As healthcare providers, we recognize the flaws in the system but feel powerless to change them. Government entities heavily regulate the way we are allowed to work and we feel as though we are at the mercy of the whims of policy makers. The limitations and frustrations that government regulations place on our practices are a key component of dissatisfaction among medical providers and they leave us feeling like we are being swept along in the mess our system has become, struggling to stay afloat.

While modern-day politicians and organizations like the Centers for Medicare and Medicaid Services (CMS) shoulder much of the blame for the frustration healthcare professionals experience, the reality is that our system is structured based on a series of decisions that were made long before CMS came into existence. There was never a master healthcare plan for Americans, but rather a collection of responsive decisions, actions, and incidents that shaped the way healthcare delivery looks in the United States today. Business models adopted early on by hospitals and insurance companies, competition among employers, lobbying by professional organizations, and government entities all played a role in creating our current healthcare landscape.

Breaking out of the toxic cycle in which so many medical practices find themselves depends on acknowledging the events that got us to where we are today. A greater understanding of the history of our healthcare system allows practices to shield providers from many of the problems our healthcare system creates, thus increasing employee satisfaction, the success of practice management, and employment relationships, and ultimately improving productivity.

HOW DID WE GET TO WHERE WE ARE TODAY?

1700s—From Home to Hospital

The foundation of the American healthcare system was laid before the United States formally became a nation. Most medical care in the 1700s took place in the home. Private physicians made house calls, primarily to the wealthy. Those who could not afford physician care relied on home remedies concocted in the kitchen.

In 1751, Benjamin Franklin and Dr. Thomas Bond took the initial step toward bringing healthcare from the home to healthcare institutions. They founded the nation's first hospital, Pennsylvania Hospital, with the mission to "care for the sick, poor, and insane who were wandering the streets of Philadelphia".[1] Early hospitals provided a way to keep sickly immigrants off the streets and away from the public, ensuring the health and comfort of the wealthy. At their inception, hospitals were looked down upon as institutions for the poor, as the wealthy continued to pay for private physicians and receive medical care in the comfort of their own homes.

1800s—Physicians' Changing Status

The early healthcare delivery model laid in the 1700s became more structured and established in the 19th century. With these changes, coupled with advancements in medicine, physicians saw their status as a profession improve. As a result, the medical profession became a lobbying force.

Physicians organize

Poor patient outcomes related to unfounded medical practices like "bleeding," postoperative complications, and a lack of understanding of infection, landed physicians squarely on a low rung in society in the early 1800s. Americans lacked confidence in medical practitioners' abilities and often opted for home remedies rather than relying on doctors for medical care. Lackluster professional licensing standards and the absence of professional organization furthered public skepticism. As a result, physicians were poorly compensated.

Seeing an opportunity to reverse the plight of physicians, in 1847, 250 delegates met in the first formal gathering of the American Medical Association (AMA).[2] The AMA had three main goals at the time.[3]

1. Restrict the number of licensed physicians by establishing medical licensing laws to create a more favorable economic climate;

2. Replace current "proprietary" medical schools with institutions requiring more extensive training to a smaller, more select group of students; and

3. Market the legitimacy of medicine to the public by denouncing practitioners with dubious practices, eliminating them from the profession.

The AMA was largely successful in its endeavors. Prior to AMA-controlled physician licensing, for example, there was one physician for every 96 people in the United States. By 1870, there was one physician for every 622 Americans.[4] Uniform education and licensing standards along with decreased competition in the medical profession served to increase physicians' status and salaries.

Key medical advancements in healthcare delivery

With dentist William T.G. Morton's advent of anesthesia and Joseph Lister's discovery of antiseptic technique, hospitals also began to rise in authority. The middle class and wealthy increasingly opted for hospital care as many healthcare services could no longer be performed in the home. The transition of healthcare delivery away from the private physicians in the home set the stage for the tension between hospitals and private physicians we still see today.

1900–1910

The early 1900s saw the invention of the airplane, the first baseball world series, and the formation of the Ford Motor Company. Organized medicine also gained momentum during this period of innovation. Advancements in medical technology continued, and healthcare professionals rose in influence. The changing face of healthcare also brought the first glimpse of the need for assistance related to covering the cost of healthcare in the form of health insurance.

The AMA as a powerful force

Physicians' newfound status paved the way for the AMA to become a powerful lobbying force. The AMA acquired its first permanent headquarters in Chicago in 1902, a symbol of its growing influence. The organization used its momentum to push its agenda even further.

In the early 1900s, the AMA sought to raise standards for medical education to even higher levels. Its efforts were advanced by publication of the Flexner Report in 1910. Written by Abraham Flexner for the Carnegie Foundation for the Advancement of Teaching, the document called on American medical schools to establish higher admission and graduation standards and adhere to more rigorous teaching and research. Flexner also recommended strengthening state regulation of medical licensure.

As a result of their efforts and bolstered by the Flexner Report, the American Medical Association saw membership increase from about 8,000 physicians in 1900 to 70,000 in 1910. The organization represented roughly half of the country's physicians at the time.

The first attempt at health reform

Medical treatment advanced in the early 1900s. Surgeries, particularly excision of masses, appendectomies, and gynecological surgeries, became more common. Despite advances in surgery and improved patient outcomes, healthcare remained relatively basic and medical costs low. In 1900, the average American spent $5 a year on health care, the equivalent of $100 by today's standards. For most Americans, the cost of medical care wasn't a concern.

Although health care was accessible and affordable in the early 1900s, cost of care did find the national spotlight. Following President William McKinley's assassination in 1901, Vice President Theodore Roosevelt assumed the presidency. A figurehead of the progressive movement, Roosevelt centered his agenda around policies favoring the common man. As part of this agenda, Roosevelt supported the concept of universal health coverage. He argued that implementing health insurance policies would curb illness and poverty, keeping the nation strong.

Despite his efforts, Roosevelt was unsuccessful in implementing health reform at the federal level. The federal government ultimately left economic health policy issues to the states, which largely ignored them, leaving private organizations to fill in any gaps.

The beginnings of employer-based health coverage

The first signs of employer-based health coverage appeared in the early 1900s. Faced with a number of workplace hazards and the near nonexistence of healthcare facilities in the areas where they operated, railroads began to hire their own surgeons and even construct their own healthcare facilities. Railroads offset some of the overhead costs of providing medical care to workers by passing the costs on to employees in the form of a fixed payroll deduction or by scaling the cost based on salary. The employer-based health system would ultimately grow in favor, becoming the standard for health insurance in the United States.

1911–1920

Politically, progressivism maintained its hold as the social movement of the decade from 1911 to 1920. In response to industrialization, activists lobbied for social and economic reforms such as improved education, workplace safety, and women's suffrage. Healthcare was not untouched by progressives calling for increased government involvement and economic reform.

A call for universal health coverage

Progressive groups lobbied for universal health coverage in the early 1900s. Germany and a number of other European countries had established social health insurance programs and progressives fought to bring a similar model to the United States.[5] The progressive proposal for universal health coverage was met with controversy; groups such as the AMA opposed the proposition.

Ultimately, the political climate, rather than organizational feuds, derailed health insurance policy efforts. In 1917, the U.S. entered World War I. Fear of socialism and communism as a result of the war steered federal health coverage out of Americans' favor.

The AMA's solid control of the medical profession

In 1914, the AMA solidified its monopoly over medical education when the organization developed standards for hospital internships. To be eligible for licensure, physicians were permitted to train exclusively at hospitals on an approved list. Effectively, the new standards awarded the AMA control over the number of spots available to physicians in training. Tight control of the number of medical students not only raised standards for the medical profession, but also kept the number of practicing physicians in the country artificially low, further inflating physician salaries.

1921–1930

Reeling from World War I, policy makers paid little attention to healthcare in the 1920s. Concerning trends in healthcare stirred in the background, however. Medical advancements like the discovery of insulin pushed healthcare spending higher. The use of hospitals became commonplace, further propelling costs upward. The few attempts to change health policy in the 1920s fizzled out as agreements could not be reached and attention was diverted to post-war recovery.

Changes in healthcare delivery

Hospitals rose in popularity in the 1920s and began marketing themselves as sites for care of much more than terminal illness. Recognizing that such services were financially out of reach of many patients, they developed innovative ways to help cover the cost of care. Baylor University Hospital was a leader in the trend and offered insurance-like plans. One such plan covered the cost of hospital visits for public school teachers in exchange for a monthly payment of 50 cents. Until this time, hospitals had always billed patients directly for services provided. The Baylor Hospital plan laid the foundation for future nonprofit Blue Cross plans and ultimately the third-party payer system as a whole.

1931–1940

The onset of the Great Depression in 1929 brought a renewed emphasis to offering government-funded benefits to Americans, redirecting attention to health insurance policy. Unregulated, an increasing number of hospitals charged exorbitant fees for services. Rising costs of medical care now left both poor and middle-income Americans unable to afford healthcare.

Another failed attempt at federal health policy

In the midst of economic crisis, the President's Committee on Economic Security under Franklin D. Roosevelt drafted the Social Security Act of 1935. The act was an attempt to curb poverty and unemployment by generating an array of assistance programs for struggling Americans. There was considerable support among politicians and the public for the inclusion of health benefits as part of the act. The AMA, however, continued to voice strong opposition to federal health benefits, declaring that such a plan would increase bureaucracy and limit doctors' autonomy. Physicians stood to lose if hospitals negotiated doctors' payments. So, despite concerns over the increasing cost of healthcare, when the bill was passed, it omitted healthcare-related legislation.

Private health insurance gains traction

In the wake of the Great Depression, hospitals were desperate to ensure payment from patients. Hospital revenues decreased as patients were unable to pay their bills and sought care at government-run institutions. One solution to the problem was to create insurance plans similar to those sold by Baylor University Hospital. Plans sold by single hospitals generated competition, so hospitals came together under the American Hospital Association (AHA), forming networks for health insurance plans. Each health insurance plan had a defined territory, reducing potentially harmful competition among hospital members. The health insurance model was a prepayment model rather than the reimbursement model we see today. In 1939, these hospital plans combined, adopting the Blue Cross name and logo.

By the end of the 1930s, approximately half of the states had passed legislation approving plans for hospital services like those of Blue Cross. Tensions between new insurance companies and the AHA rose, as meeting the needs of individual hospitals and Blue Cross were often in conflict.

1941–1950

The 1940s were perhaps the most influential years in the development of health insurance policy in the United States. The decade also saw the formation of the physician assistant profession, ringing in the age of midlevel medical providers.

Post-war health policy attempts

Shortly after taking office in 1945, President Harry Truman called for mandatory health insurance for all Americans. Health insurance plans would be funded by payroll deductions and cover the cost of medical and hospital services.

Entangled in World War II, mandatory health insurance legislation was written off by Americans as socialism. Furthermore, the American Medical Association claimed that Truman's plan would make doctors "slaves." The AMA was so passionate in its opposition of Truman's agenda that in 1945, the organization spent $1.5 million on lobbying efforts and assessed each of their members a $25 fee to assist in compulsory health insurance resistance efforts. Truman's plan died in a Congressional committee.

Employer-based health insurance takes shape

While Truman was unsuccessful at passing federal health insurance legislation, the private health insurance market rapidly expanded in the 1940s. During World War II, the government mandated wage controls for employers. Such controls placed a ceiling on wages in an attempt to curb inflation.

To compensate for wage controls and compete for qualified employees, employers began to offer health insurance coverage as a non-wage incentive. Health insurance became a popular fringe benefit offered by employers to attract employees in a climate when providing higher salaries was not an option. This was the beginning of the employer-based system we have today.

Health insurance plans administered by hospitals themselves also rapidly gained popularity. In 1938, only 300,000 Americans were covered by such policies. By 1946, more than 6 million Americans had purchased commercial insurance.[6]

Midlevel providers emerge

The origins of the physician assistant profession also took root as a result of World War II fallout. An insufficient number of physicians in the battlefield forced medical leaders to look for a way to meet the increasing need for healthcare among soldiers in a timely manner. Two schools of medical training were developed. These institutions offered modified physician training programs preparing healthcare providers in an accelerated timeframe.

1951–1960

Few legislative changes were made to federal health policy in the 1950s as Americans diverted attention to the Korean War. During the war, however, commercial and employer-based health insurance plans gained further traction and expand their offerings.

Motivation for employer-based health insurance grows

Employer-based health insurance coverage became even more popular in the 1950s with Congress' new IRS code, the Code of 1954. The new tax law mandated that health insurance premiums paid by employers were tax exempt. Now, employers had even more incentive to offer the popular benefit.[7] Prior to 1950, only 12.2% of Blue Cross plans received employer contributions; by 1950, employers paid for about half of the "gross cost" of health insurance for employees and 30% of the cost of covering dependents.

As health insurance plans grew in popularity and expanded coverage options, insurers were careful to mitigate risk to the company. Individuals with preexisting conditions were excluded from plans, keeping the cost of health insurance reasonable and the risk for health insurance companies low. As a result, the elderly and those who are very sick had difficulty finding coverage.[6]

1961–1970

The 1960s proved to be a significant contrast to the health reform-free years of the 1950s as problems with health insurance plans arose. Life expectancy was increasing as a result of medical advancement. New treatments were costlier, further increasing the cost of healthcare. So, insurance companies raised premiums. Very few elderly individuals had health insurance at all, as it was not a prevalent benefit offered nor a necessity during their lifetimes.

Democrats planned to intervene to help the poor and elderly by expanding the Social Security Act of 1935. The proposed expansion would provide comprehensive health coverage for individuals age 65 and older through a new program: Medicare.

Many organizations opposed government involvement in healthcare, and the American Medical Association was a noteworthy party in opposition. In 1961, the organization launched a lobbying effort against Medicare titled Operation Coffee Cup. Ronald Reagan, whose father-in-law was serving as president of the AMA, played a key role in the operation in which 3,000 wives of physicians invited friends and neighbors over for coffee and played a record of Reagan speaking out against socialism and Medicare's creation.[8] The lobbying effort proved temporarily successful; the bill was struck down by the Senate in 1961 under the Kennedy administration.

The tide, however, eventually turned against the AMA. Despite opposition, President Lyndon B. Johnson was successful in passing the Social Security Act of 1965, which included the creation of Medicare and Medicaid. Originally, Medicare included only Part A, hospital insurance, and Part B, medical insurance. Medicaid assisted states in covering the cost of healthcare for the poor and disabled. In honor of Truman's earlier work toward a government-funded health insurance program, Johnson awarded the former president and his wife Bess the first Medicare cards in 1966.[9]

There were no government think tanks estimating the cost of proposed legislation at the time Medicare was passed. While Congress took into account the expense of running the program, it was not central to Congressional Medicare debate. Healthcare expenditures as a percentage of gross domestic product rose sharply following the implementation of the Social Security Act of 1965.[10]

Medical profession moves toward specialization

Another trend that had been slowly rearing its head in healthcare emerged in force: physician specialization. By the 1960s, 69% of physicians were specialists. In 1964, just 19% of medical school graduates entered general practice, down from 47% in 1900. Given the expansion of medical skills and procedures in recent years, medical students expressed concern that mastery of general practice covered too much content. Family practice also suffered from a lack of prestige among emerging specialties and advancements in surgery.[11] The rise in the number of specialty physicians further drove up the cost of medical care and facilitated the development of a disconnected healthcare system.

Nurse practitioner profession established

Physicians across the country had begun to unofficially mentor and collaborate with experienced nurses, teaching them to increase their roles within their medical practices. Meanwhile, the increasing specialization of physicians created a primary care shortage in many areas of the country.

Noting this trend, in 1965, nurse Loretta Ford and physician Henry Silver partnered to found the nation's first pediatric nurse practitioner program at the University of Colorado's School of Medicine and Nursing. The goal of the new program was to expand the role of the public health nurse with an emphasis on health promotion and preventative health.

Ford received pushback from both the nursing and medical communities. Nursing leaders expressed concern that the expansion made the nursing role "ambiguous." Physician organizations opposed the concept, arguing that nurses should not function without direct physician supervision. In a 2011 CNN interview, Ford stated "There was great concern, I think, that the kind of direction that we were taking was much more medical than nursing," a sentiment that remains to some extent today.

Initially the nurse practitioner role was ill-defined and informal. No standard certification, licensure, or legal standards regulated the profession. Nurse practitioners increasingly legitimized their role in the medical field in the 1970s by documenting patient satisfaction with their care and demonstrating their ability to provide primary care services in areas that did not have access to healthcare.

1971–1980

The cost of healthcare increased exponentially following the passage of Medicare and Medicaid. Healthcare costs had risen from 4% of the federal budget in 1965 to 11% by 1973, a staggering jump. Millions of Americans under the age of 65 were still uninsured and unable to afford medical services. In an effort to stabilize healthcare expenditure, President Richard Nixon signed into law the Health Maintenance Organization Act of 1973.

The Act provided federal funding to insurance plans in which coverage was prepaid in fixed amounts, and at rates less expensive than individual rates. The thinking at the time was that implementing HMOs on a wider scale would facilitate the delivery of healthcare within a more efficient model. These plans, for example, incentivized preventative care, theoretically cutting long-term medical costs. By 1996, 74% of American employees were participating in HMO insurance plans.[12]

President Nixon hoped to further extend his influence over healthcare with his proposed Comprehensive Health Insurance Plan (CHIP), which called for universal health insurance coverage, funded partially by employers. Congress seemed poised to reach an agreement regarding the expansive health insurance legislation. Watergate hearings, however, interrupted the Congressional health insurance debate, overshadowing health reform.

Despite efforts to quell the rise of health costs in the 1970s through HMOs, the cost of providing healthcare to Americans continued to soar. In 1970, Americans spent $74.9 billion on medical care, a figure that rose to $212 billion by 1979.[12] Ultimately, Nixon's Health Maintenance Organization Act was not enough to turn the tide of the rising cost of healthcare.

1981–1990

Fueled by technological advances in medicine and increased ability to treat and manage chronic disease, healthcare costs continued to escalate rapidly in the 1980s. The disturbing trend prompted even further interest in HMOs, so much so that enrollment in HMOs expanded from 9 million in 1980 to 33 million by 1990. Capitation, in which participating physicians received a set amount for each patient insured regardless of the patient's usage of the system, was promoted as a method by which HMOs might contain health costs, replacing the fee-for-service model.

Despite their popularity, HMOs did not cut healthcare costs as much as anticipated, propagating other types of managed care plans such as Preferred Provider Organizations, or PPOs. As a whole, managed care plans curbed healthcare costs by incentivizing physicians to select less costly plans of care, reviewing the medical necessity of procedures, and limiting the number of inpatient hospital admissions.[6]

Unintended consequences of managed care

One consequence of the popularity of managed care plans was the consolidation of healthcare entities. As part of managed care, insurance companies negotiated with a limited number of healthcare providers and facilities. So, hospitals aggregated and bought out private physician practices in an effort to increase bargaining power. With fewer healthcare organizations in the market, hospitals were able to strike more favorable deals with insurance companies.

Ultimately, managed care plans did help curb healthcare costs as they gained popularity in the 1980s. The effect, however, was not substantial enough to serve as the ultimate solution to making healthcare affordable for Americans. The political stage was set for another massive health spending overhaul.

1991–2000

While managed care insurance plans helped curb the cost of healthcare as they gained popularity, costs continued to rise. The cost of healthcare increased at double the rate of inflation, and the cost of Medicare also grew at double the rate of inflation as it had every year since 1966. Politicians realized the need for reform.

Hillarycare

After his election, President Bill Clinton centered much of his political agenda around healthcare, appointing his wife, Hillary, as head of the effort. Consequently, the "managed competition" plan, formally titled the Health Security Act, became known as "Hillarycare."

Clinton's plan called for universal health insurance coverage, an employer and individual mandate, as well as government regulation of competition among insurance companies. Ultimately, the bill lacked popularity in Congress and did not garner enough support to pass.

Health reform affects physician reimbursement

Although sweeping health reform efforts on a national legislative level were once again defeated during the Clinton administration, policy makers were successful in instituting change on a smaller level, namely in the way physicians were reimbursed by Medicare. At the time, physicians billed Medicare based on the guidelines of a "usual, customary, and reasonable" (UCR) charge. More or less, this charge was whatever doctors decided to bill for their services.

Medicare's reimbursement rates for services billed under this system were determined based on a weighted average of what physicians in the same community billed for the same service. Physicians billing under the UCR system were reimbursed at much higher rates for performing procedures and surgeries than for other types of patient care.

As the cost of healthcare continued to rise, Congress sought to implement a new system that would decrease Medicare's long-term spending growth rate and divide payments to physicians more equitably. Disparities between reimbursement rates for procedures and other forms of patient care fueled the demand for change.

The Resource-Based Relative Value Scale (RBRVS) was the solution. The new reimbursement scale, passed as part of the Omnibus Reconciliation Act of 1989, was implemented in 1992. One goal of the new system was to correct the imbalance of reimbursement between specialty physicians and primary care providers. The system used what it called Relative Value Units, or RVUs, to quantify the amount of work, practice overhead, and malpractice risk associated with physician services to set reimbursement rates.

In the first six years of its implementation, the RBRVS system saw payments to family practice physicians increase by 36% and payments to specialty physicians decrease by 18%. RVUs were also used by private insurance companies to measure physician productivity. Since its implementation, the RVU model has undergone several adjustments, but it remains as the standard for physician reimbursement today.

2001–2010

Medicare's fiscal sustainability was increasingly called into question in the early 2000s. Doubts about the efficacy of the employer-based health insurance system also began to mount. Increasing attention to the cost of healthcare and Medicare's perilous state made health reform a natural focus early in the 2008 presidential campaign. The collapse of the housing market and economic downturn of the United States, however, soon overshadowed healthcare in campaign speeches. Once again, health reform was pushed to the legislative back burner.

Despite a temporary shift in focus, in February 2009, newly elected President Barack Obama declared that "healthcare reform cannot wait, it must not wait, it will not wait another year." He created the Office of Health Reform to launch his administrative effort to address the nation's healthcare woes, holding its first healthcare summit in March of the same year.

Bitter controversy surrounded proposed healthcare legislation in both the House and Senate. Allegations that the health reform bill included "death panels" that would decide whether people would live or die, for example, divided the public and Congress on President Obama's bill. Ultimately, the legislation garnered support, and Congress passed the Patient Protection and Affordable Care Act, on March, 23, 2010.

The most notable provision in the Affordable Care Act was the mandate that all individuals attain health insurance by 2014, either through an employer or in the individual market. Individuals without access to affordable health coverage through employment could purchase insurance with the aid of federal subsidies through new health insurance "exchanges."

WHERE WE ARE TODAY

Ultimately, the government's attempts to regulate and control the cost of healthcare in our country have placed immense pressure on healthcare providers. Constantly adapting to changes in healthcare legislation and health insurance trends has left providers feeling fatigued. Government intervention in the system complicates day-to-day interactions between patients and providers. The outlook of healthcare careers lies in the hands of policy makers, outside the control of individual providers themselves.

Physician reimbursement with the RVU system stands out as one such policy that significantly impacts the daily life of healthcare providers. RVUs have become the benchmark for reimbursement and are used by nearly all third-party payers. Essentially, this system turns healthcare providers from patient-focused medical professionals into salespeople. It compensates for the quantity of care provided rather than its quality. Under this system, healthcare providers find themselves in a place of moral compromise. Making the best medical decision for a patient doesn't always pay. Selling more services, procedures, surgeries, and ancillary services does.

Employers in the healthcare sector often tie RVU reimbursement directly to providers' paychecks, further reinforcing the shortcomings of this system. The result is pressure to "sell" and to provide more "care" to patients regardless of medical necessity. Quickly, healthcare providers become disillusioned, workplace cultures are poisoned with competition and dissatisfaction—a recipe for employee turnover and burnout.

While individual medical providers and employers may be relatively powerless to change the healthcare system on a national scale, employers do have the power to insulate providers from the negative effects that naturally result from working within a flawed system. By shielding healthcare providers from the pressures created by our healthcare system, employers enable providers to focus on patient care. Allowing providers to focus on patient care effectively fosters satisfaction of both providers and patients, ultimately increasing productivity.

REFERENCES

1. Penn Medicine. In the beginning: The story of the creation of the mation's first hospital. Penn Medicine Web site. (n.d.). www.uphs.upenn.edu/paharc/features/creation.html. Accessed November 15, 2016.
2. The Editors of Encyclopædia Britannica. American Medical Association (AMA). www.britannica.com/topic/American-Medical-Association. Accessed November 13, 2016.
3. Hamowy R. The early development of medical licensing laws in the United States, 1875-1900. *J Libert Stud.* 1979;3(1):73-119. Retrieved November 13, 2016, from https://mises.org/library/early-development-medical-licensing-laws-united-states-1875-1900
4. Loker, TW. *The history and evolution of healthcare in America: The untold backstory of where we've been, where we are, and why healthcare needs reform.* Bloomington, IN: iUniverse:2012.
5. Hoffman, B. Health care reform and social movements in the United States. *Am J. Public Health.* 2003 January; 93(1):5-85.
6. Jost, T.S. History of health insurance in the United States. In: *The Encyclopedia of Health Economics.* London: Elsevier: 2014.
7. Employer-Sponsored Health Insurance and Health Reform. The National Bureau of Economic Research Web site. www.nber.org/bah/2009no2/w14839.htmlRetrieved November 20, 2016, from

8. Hyman, DA. *Medicare meets mephistopheles*. Washington, D.C.: Cato Institute: 2006.

9. President Lyndon B. Johnson Signs Medicare Bill. Harry S. Truman Library & Museum Web site. https://www.trumanlibrary.org/anniversaries/medicarebill.htm. Accessed November 19, 2016.

10. National Health Insurance—A Brief History Of Reform Efforts In The U.S. The Henry J. Kaiser Family Foundation Web site. http://kff.org/health-reform/issue-brief/national-health-insurance-a-brief-history-of. Accessed November 22, 2016.

11. American Board of Family Medicine: History of the Specialty. The American Board of Family Medicine Web site. www.theabfm.org/about/history.aspx. Accessed November 13, 2016.

12. Health Maintenance Organization Act of 1973 Primary Source. eNotes Web site. www.enotes.com/topics/health-maintenance-organization-act-1973. Accessed November 13, 2016.

CHAPTER 10

In the End—Doing What's Best for Your Practice and Employees

What frustrates you in your practice and what you can do about it

For many physicians, the growing burden of government involvement in healthcare proves to be a significant stressor. Keeping up with the latest requirements from CMS and private insurance companies not only increases practice overhead, but tends to be a soul-sucking task. For other physicians, a lack of work-life balance takes the cake. Early mornings, late evenings, and taking call at all hours of the night leaves you a slave to your practice. In yet other cases, physicians are simply fed up with lack of time to devote to professional tasks they enjoy, such as academic research or a particular subset of patients.

What would it be like if you could revive the altruistic vision you once had for your career as an MD, at least in some sense? How would your outlook on life and your career change if you could offload some of these practice burdens you carry? Practices across the country are doing just that with nurse practitioners and physician assistants.

As a practice, you have options when it comes to employing NPs and PAs. Advanced practice providers are uniquely equipped to fill flexible roles. Practices across the country of all kinds are developing models that solve the problems faced in their specific setting with these providers.

While some medical associations shun midlevel providers, concerned with competition in the healthcare market, others are recognizing this value that NPs and PAs have to offer. Urologists, for example, have had such success integrating NPs and PAs into their patient care model that the American Urological Association released a consensus statement supporting the integration of advanced practice providers into these specialized practices.[1]

One example of success within the specialty comes from Urology Associates, P.C. in Nashville, Tennessee, a 32-physician group that employs 12 midlevel providers. Integrating NPs and PAs into the group's staffing model has allowed for the creation of new service lines in the practice that not only serve middle Tennessee's patients, but also translate into additional lines of revenue. In one such endeavor, a women's health nurse practitioner hired by the practice was foundational in opening a clinic focused on female sexual dysfunction—a service largely ignored by other clinics in the area. She forged relationships with local primary care practices to generate a referral stream and now manages the majority of new patients referred to the practice.[2]

Advanced practice providers also have helped maintain the practice's high patient volume while simultaneously allowing physicians to focus on areas of the specialty that yield the highest reimbursement rates, such as surgeries and specialized procedures.

Similar success stories prevail in the hospitalist world. At Rush University Medical Center in Chicago, for example, Dr. Suparna Dutta explains that advanced practice providers have taken on a significant level of responsibility on the hospital floor. One of the facility's 16-patient inpatient services, for example, assigns half of patients to NPs and PAs while the attending physician manages the eight most complex cases. The system allows care to take place in an efficient manner, maximizing the strengths and training of each provider.

The path to seamless utilization of advanced practice providers at Rush University Medical Center took time and a plan, Dr. Dutta cautions. "At first, we had two APPs, fresh out of school, functioning as residents, rounding together and doing work like calling consults and calling orders in. As APPs improved and we grew the service, they were able to expand into more fulfilling roles with more autonomy with their own patients where they have first crack at making decisions with oversight and backup as needed," she tells *ACP Hospitalist*.[3]

In yet another clinical environment, physician J. Scott Litton relates his success with hiring nurse practitioners. Dr. Litton opened a private clinic in his hometown of Pennington Gap, Virginia. His patient panel grew rapidly given his roots in the area, and Dr. Litton was faced with a difficult decision: stop accepting new patients or take the risk of expanding. Seventeen months after founding his practice, he hired a nurse practitioner and hasn't looked back. The NP not only covered acute same-day visits, but also offloaded some of Dr. Litton's patient volume, allowing him to continue to accept new patients—about one or two per day.

Patient satisfaction soared with the addition of the new provider and volume continued to grow. The move proved so effective that four years later, he brought a second nurse practitioner on board. Dr. Litton's recipe for success? "Remember that when adding a midlevel provider to your practice, have a very rigid protocol in place for the midlevel to follow so that the care that is provided can be easily supervised and monitored by the physician(s)," he advises.[4]

Not only does the career outlook of physicians stand to improve with the implementation of advanced practice providers, it does so in a cost-effective manner. A study by the University to Texas Southwestern Medical Center, for example, found that the overhead costs of physician assistant employment were significantly lower than those for physicians. In fact, researchers estimated that a PA can boost revenues by $30,000 or more in overhead savings alone.[5] Similarly, a study conducted in the HMO setting found that adding a nurse practitioner to a practice can nearly double patient volume, resulting in a $1.65 million revenue increase per 100,000 enrollees.[6]

BENEFITING YOUR PRACTICE

Nurse practitioners and physician assistants can be an asset to your practice when it comes to practice efficiencies, work-life balance, and generating revenue. As the anecdotes above caution, you must have a framework in place for the midlevel provider role. In order for midlevel providers to thrive and contribute to your practice you must commit to:

1. Understand the role of nurse practitioners and physician assistants;
2. Recognize that midlevel providers are not salespeople; and
3. Provide transparency around hiring and compensation.

Without these principles in place, practices limit the benefits they stand to gain with advanced practice providers.

Understand the Role of Nurse Practitioners and Physician Assistants

Midlevel providers don't go to medical school. This seems like an obvious point, yet too many practices expect these NPs and PAs to perform like physicians without supplemental training. Embarrassingly, my nurse practitioner program at a highly regarded university didn't even teach family nurse practitioners how to read ECGs or perform minor office procedures. These essential practice skills were left to be learned on the job.

Training and mentoring are essential for nurse practitioners and physician assistants in your practice. Without them, at best, you will fail to maximize the benefits these providers have to offer. At worst, you compromise the quality of care in your practice, increasing liability and risking negative patient outcomes. Practices must implement a structure for the training, mentoring, and education of midlevel providers.

Recognize That Midlevel Providers Are Not Salespeople

The government has turned healthcare providers into salespeople. The more we "do," the fatter our paychecks. Advanced practice providers, however, did not enter the healthcare profession to sell services. Shield your NPs and PAs from government whims by compensating them on a salaried basis. Not only does this mitigate potential conflict and mistrust in your practice, it increases provider satisfaction so that they stick around for the long haul.

Furthermore, salaried (or hourly) compensation gives your practice greater flexibility in the way you structure midlevel provider staffing to maximize efficiency and revenue in your practice. Productivity-based compensation, in contrast, leaves midlevel providers at risk for burnout. It creates a competitive work environment and additional pressure adding to the stress of healthcare employment.

Provide Transparency Around Hiring and Compensation

Rather than incentivizing advanced practice providers with productivity-based compensation, encourage improved performance with a clearly outlined compensation structure.

Share this early in the hiring process so it's apparent to NPs and PAs what they must do to become top earners in your practice. This allows your practice to reward metrics that are most important to the group, rather than tying you to the government's pay-for-performance system.

Decide how your practice would best benefit from hiring NPs and PAs. Build these responsibilities into your compensation structure so midlevel providers prioritize these responsibilities. Not only does this ensure that your visions for employment are aligned, it provides a framework for upward mobility in the practice, a major contributor to job satisfaction in what can become a stagnant role. Outline what growth within your practice looks like and stick to your plan.

The benefits midlevel providers stand to provide come with responsibility. If you hire NPs and PAs, be prepared for to play a managerial role in your practice. Anticipate how this will affect physicians' ability to see patients and decide on a structure for training and mentoring that works best for your practice. The time you put in at the front end will pay off in a successful employment relationship, allowing you to maximize the benefits that working with nurse practitioners and physician assistants has to offer.

REFERENCES

1. Gonzalez CM, Brand T, Koncz L, et al. AUA Consensus Statement on Advanced Practice Providers: Executive Summary. *Urology Practice*. 2015;2(5).
2. Concepcion R. Working with APPs: Best practices from a successful practice. *Urology Times*. August 1, 2015. Retrieved February 21, 2017, from http://urologytimes.modernmedicine.com/urology-times/news/working-apps-best-practices-successful-practice?page=0,1
3. D'Arrigo T. Getting the most from advanced practice providers. *ACP Hospitalist*. December 2016. Retrieved February 21, 2017, from www.acphospitalist.org/archives/2016/12/advanced-practice-providers.htm
4. Litton JS. (2015, April 15). How midlevel providers can enhance your practice. *Physicians Practice*. April 15, 2015. Retrieved February 21, 2017, from www.physicianspractice.com/blog/how-midlevel-providers-can-enhance-your-practice
5. Jones PE, & Cawley JF. (1994). Physician assistants and health system reform. Clinical capabilities, practice activities, and potential roles. *JAMA*, 1994 Apr 27;271(16):1266-172.
6. Burl J, Bonner A, Rao M, & Khan A. (1998). Geriatric nurse practitioners in long-term care: demonstration of effectiveness in managed care. *J Am Geriatr Soc*. 1998 Apr;46(4):506-10.

www.ingramcontent.com/pod-product-compliance
Lightning Source LLC
Chambersburg PA
CBHW081545220326
41598CB00036B/6576